18110

Hyperemesis Gravidarum

A BAME Mother's Story

RACHAEL BUABENG

ISBN: 978-0-9956641-5-9

Cover design by Chaneen Saliee. All rights reserved.
Edited by Dalitso Tembo
JLG Publishing

Printed in the United Kingdom

DEDICATION

Dedicated to the two beautiful blessings that are my babies on earth and my Angel in the sky who taught me to always look for the rainbow.

Thanks be to God for motherhood!

CONTENTS

ACKNOWLEDGEMENTS

ACKNOWLEDGMENTS

I want to acknowledge the NHS staff especially, those at Homerton Hospital, Hackney, UK. Namely, I want to thank my midwife Theodora Tsikplornu who was exceptionally supportive throughout both my pregnancies. Theodora empowered me despite my sickness to take care of me and the baby. She attentively listened to my challenges and equipped me with enough knowledge to maintain my health and deal with cultural challenges. I will forever remember you and the personalised care you gave me.

~

To my friends and family - I thank you for not judging me and thinking I was making this thing up. Thank you for the support and love you all showed me throughout my pregnancy journeys.

Belinda and Kweku, thank you for always offering me your sofa to crash on.

P.S. Thank you all for standing up for me when everyone and their gran wanted to tell me how to manage hyperemesis gravidarum.

~

To my husband - THANK YOU. I will never know what ran through your mind when you heard the words hyperemesis gravidarum, but I thank you for never letting your own feelings affect the care you gave me. I thank you for always buying what I wanted to eat, although you bought way too much of each thing. Thank you for all the times you slept in the hospital chair and for your patience throughout our journey.

~

Finally, thank you to my children. For all the times our plans got cancelled because of me being sick because I was growing your siblings, thank you Amaryah for your patience. Ava-Rose at only two years old, you were able to help Mummy while I was vomiting. Thank you for being such an angel and a protector to me. You may never remember the time when Mummy was sick, but you were very helpful and always brought me my bucket.
Love you!

FOREWORDS

FOREWORDS

It's been a long time since reading a book that has brought me to both tears of joy and gladness while experiencing moments of self-forgiveness at the same time. I have experienced Hyperemesis Gravidarum (HG) during the pregnancy of my first son, which was a very challenging experience. I went on to have another experience with my second son but, this time around it was an even more difficult experience as I became a single mother with a toddler and I had work-related issues to add.

Thankfully, I was fortunate to have had some knowledge about HG as I am a qualified Midwife and a Health Visitor by profession but, there were many moments I just needed reassurance from somebody who had experienced the untold truths of what I was going through. Some of those truths mentioned are the need to carry heavy pads and spare underwear in your bag, which in my case it was actually baby nappies I needed (I never thought I would ever have to discuss this in my lifetime but here I am letting you know what I needed at the time).

Reading this book brings joy knowing that the author has taken the step to raise awareness of these unspoken experiences that women with HG go through. I am glad that a woman somewhere can find this book at a time she most needs a Mum-friend who has been through it and be reassured. The author has vast knowledge in the teaching profession, she is someone who has survived HG a number of times and she is very passionate about supporting other women through her words of encouragement, which makes her the best candidate to write this story.

A BAME Mother's Story is a treasure to a mother who is at the crossroads, asking the questions, knocking on the doors of others around her but does not find that person she can truly relate to, the one that can open up the door and let her into the insights of the reality of what she is going through as a result of HG. I am a true believer in gaining knowledge that will help to make an informed decision for yourself in any given situation.

One way I have come to realise over the years of my personal and professional experience is that knowledge gained through an authentic and relatable story that is based on a person's life experience can be the miracle-pill that saves someone from the road of self-pity, self-sabotage or even depression.

This book vividly describes the events that led up to the author being diagnosed with HG in the simplest form for any reader with no medical background to understand. The author also uses factual guidance that is usually offered by medical practitioners such as medication to be taken as prescribed, which can easily be overlooked by a woman with HG as she does not want to feel like an incompetent Mum-to-be or even feel judged by those around her.

I adore how she has included some culturally relatable humour in the encouragement sections to share practical tips that equip the reading mother in order to safeguard herself and her unborn baby. I want to applaud the author for taking the time to outline some of the challenges that a woman with HG goes through in such detail as it can be something that most survivors try to not remember as it can be a traumatic period. The author highly recommends access to therapy especially for women that experience HG as mental health is paramount and making sure if the woman feels unheard to make sure to speak out and seek further advice.

Taking into consideration that every experience is different from woman to woman. I can say this book has definitely brought a lot of relatable experiences to light for me. I am honoured to have had this opportunity to write this foreword for this book as someone who has sat on both sides of the table as the professional offering advice to another woman who is pregnant and the other as a client/patient who needed someone to just understand the challenges I was facing and I didn't come across a book such as this one at those times. I wholeheartedly hope that the woman that reads this book will feel reassured and connected to the author as a friend who has walked a similar journey and only wants nothing more than to support others while building a much-needed awareness of HG in the BAME community.

Belinda Bvute
Midwife,
Health Visitor& Founder of Ambitious Mums

ADDITIONAL FOREWORD

An additional foreword from a HG survivor and Midwife based in Ghana:

I grew up in a society where Hyperemesis Gravidarum (HG) is not recognised as a disease despite its severity and effect on the pregnant woman and her baby. I first heard of this big term in Midwifery school.

The author of this book and I met on social media, yes on Instagram. For years I was a secret admirer who admired her work mainly because of her passion for mothers and mothers-to-be. Her passion is evident in the events she organises for mums to get away from all the beautiful chaos of their daily life to unwind, share ideas and come up with ways to make this journey of motherhood easier. This goes a long way to help their mental health. As an experienced midwife of 10 years, working with pregnant women and new mothers with a similar passion as hers is inspiring, empowering and encouraging.

Being an HG survivor myself (yes, I call it that because not all women live to tell their story), this book speaks to me on a personal level. I have had HG in two pregnancies, and one of them resulted in a miscarriage. The second which I was able to carry to term was filled with ups and downs as there were days where I wished I wasn't pregnant. This was not because I didn't want the pregnancy, far from that, I wanted it badly. In fact, I fought for it but the feeling of always being sick, despair and impending doom was enough to mess with my head at times. Yes, even with my years of experience as a midwife. Would it have been better if I had this book? Oh yes.

The author has suffered this condition in all her pregnancies, and she goes out of her way to recount her experiences and that is not the only thing that makes this book worthy of reading it is the vivid picture she paints. If you are a woman going through it, it would feel like she is telling your story, each chapter comes with an encouragement section where she discusses what helped her get through mentally and physically. That is the part I wished I had and that is my favourite part.

Her passion for building awareness for almost everything related to women and motherhood doesn't make this book ordinary. The advice is a real-life application of what worked for her and other women. She didn't leave any aspect out, even topics such as intimacy. She takes you through her journey whilst discussing the physiological, emotional, social, economical and cultural effect of HG woman with the lessons learnt. Each chapter offers what can be done to help, especially coming from a society and culture that has a mental picture of how a perfect pregnancy must be, against which all pregnancies are measured.

The loved ones and support systems of women suffering HG do not have the knowledge to attribute meaning to HG symptoms, thereby criticising HG sufferers, increasing the feeling of self-doubt, stress and anxiety. As a professional I often witness first-hand women reporting symptoms of HG, even in the emergency room having their symptoms minimised by hospital staff and therefore, are delayed getting care till things get out of hand. Therefore, this book helps increase the wider awareness of the impact of HG and offers comfort for pregnant women suffering from HG and helps HG survivors get closure.

Jocelyne Marina Agbeko
Midwifery officer, Midwifery Tutor
Founder; Pregnancy Matters Ghana

WHAT IS HYPEREMESIS GRAVIDARUM?

WHAT IS HYPEREMESIS GRAVIDARUM?

Hyperemesis Gravidarum (HG) is severe nausea, vomiting, rapid weight loss, malnutrition and dehydration due to excessive vomiting. Unlike *'morning sickness'* HG puts both mother and baby at risk as it can cause an inability to eat as normal due to the feeling of severe nausea and excessive vomiting. This feeling can occur up to 50 times a day, and as a result, it can significantly interfere with the daily life of the pregnant woman. [1]

HG typically starts between the fourth and seventh weeks of gestation and peaks in the ninth week. For 90% of pregnant women with HG, the experience continues up until the 20th week. [2]

CAUSE

The cause for HG is unknown; however, there have been speculations by experts that it could be linked to the changing hormones in the body. Previous research in HG has also suggested that there is a link between HG and genetics. There is also evidence to suggest that if you have had HG in a previous pregnancy, then there is a higher chance of you having it again in your next pregnancy compared to women who have never had it before. [3]

TREATMENT

There are a few treatments for HG that can be used in pregnancy including in the 'first twelve weeks,' to improve the symptoms such as antiemetic (anti-sickness) drugs, vitamins B6 and B12 and in extreme cases steroids.[4]

---

[1]Fejzo, M.S., Trovik, J., Grooten, I.J., Sridharan, K., Roseboom, T.J., Vikanes, Å., Painter, R.C. and Mullin, P.M. (2019). Nausea and vomiting of pregnancy and hyperemesis gravidarum. *Nature Reviews Disease Primers*, 5(1).

[2]NHS Choices (2019). *Severe vomiting in pregnancy- Your pregnancy and baby guide.* [online] Available at: https://www.nhs.uk/conditions/pregnancy-and-baby/severe-vomiting-in-pregnancy-hyperemesis-gravidarum/.

[3] Koot, M.H., Grooten, I.J., van der Post, J.A.M., Bais, J.M.J., Ris-Stalpers, C., Leeflang, M.M.G., Bremer, H.A., van der Ham, D.P., Heidema, W.M., Huisjes, A., Kleiverda, G., Kuppens, S.M., van Laar, J.O.E.H., Langenveld, J., van der Made, F., van Pampus, M.G., Papatsonis, D., Pelinck, M.-J., Pernet, P.J., van Rheenen-Flach, L., Rijnders, R.J., Scheepers, H.C.J., Vogelvang, T.E., Mol, B.W., Roseboom, T.J. and Painter, R.C. (2020). Determinants of disease course and severity in hyperemesis gravidarum. *European Journal of Obstetrics &Gynecology and Reproductive Biology*, [online] 245, pp.162–167. Available at: https://www.sciencedirect.com/science/article/abs/pii/S0301211519305883 [Accessed 5 May 2020].

[4] Fiaschi, L., Nelson-Piercy, C., Deb, S., King, R. and Tata, L. (2019). Clinical management of nausea and vomiting in pregnancy and hyperemesis gravidarum across primary and secondary care: a population-based study. *BJOG: An International Journal of Obstetrics & Gynaecology*, 126(10), pp.1201–1211.

1

I'M PREGNANT!

At this point, I had been married for over a year and, knowing how much I wanted children many people were surprised that we were not pregnant yet. To be fair I was surprised too but I wasn't worried. The biggest challenge was navigating the '*aunties*' that would approach me with absolute no tact and absolutely no sense of remorse. The words '*Won't you hurry and have a baby?*' were always shouted my way. The problem for many is that some of these aunties come in the form of your mother, friend and even their husbands. Sigh.

Then finally, we are pregnant! The three pregnancy tests confirmed it, and the smile across my face said it all. I already felt different. My whole life, I always wanted to get pregnant and become a Mum. I wanted six children and I promised myself that I would do everything within my power to give my children the best life possible. Finally, my dream was slowly becoming a reality and it felt amazing.

I was overwhelmed with excitement but, as a few weeks passed, I started to experience continuous nausea, and on several occasions I had excess saliva and bouts of vomiting. My body had already started to change and, as traditions would have it, I was patiently waiting for the three-month mark before I told anyone outside of the immediate family that I was pregnant. This became increasingly difficult as by the second month of my pregnancy I was already sporting an obvious bump. As expected people began to notice and what was meant to be kept a secret for three months went straight to pot. Everyone could see something was growing in my belly plus my face had changed, and I was vomiting, which was the ultimate giveaway.

Halfway through my second month of pregnancy, I attended a thanksgiving service with my family, as you do. It took what felt like forever to get ready, but I was happy to go out to a safe space with people I loved. At this point, I didn't care what I wore as I had already been poorly and knew I was getting closer to my three-month mark. It felt like too much hassle to hide it whilst also trying to manage my vomiting. Besides I could finally wear a bodycon and have a round belly without thinking about whether I should use a 'girdle' or not.

Typical of my Ghanaian aunties, they knew I was pregnant straight away and I was immediately showered with advice. I was told not to wear heels, take it easy and most of all don't have sex yet, which of course made me cringe. These open chats took place in the car park whilst I was vomiting and only making eye contact to acknowledge them. To some this would be awful but, I was so happy to finally be free and share my pregnancy experience with my favourite aunties and cousins.

My aunts made me feel so loved and it was like I was being initiated into the new milestone of life. They were proud and happy for me, so much so that even me vomiting into the bush behind the car was a reassuring sign to them. They encouraged me and reassured me that I will be ok. They reminded me to pray about my pregnancy and remain prayerful always. My Mum was also on hand to confirm that I did vomit quite a bit which almost made my vomiting behind the car justified and that I wasn't vomiting on cue in front of family (yes as crazy as it seems that is what I thought it could look like.) I felt warm (still sicky) but very warm inside listening to them. Little did I know this would be the last family gathering I would attend for a little while.

My face slowly switched from smiling to a frown and continuous feeling of uncertainty as to when I would vomit next. I was only two months pregnant and feeling like I was on a rollercoaster every day. I continued to try to function like the other pregnant women I knew, which of course was not what I should have been doing. As time went on, I had so many questions. *'Why was I feeling so sick? What was wrong with me?'* This was supposed to be the best time of my life. I remembered that my aunties had said that nausea and vomiting in pregnancy (NVP) was normal. My Mum also always reminded me that pregnancy did come with some nausea and vomiting. She reassured me when I questioned why they call it morning sickness if I am sick at several parts of my day. The funny thing was I knew that but, I was just looking for someone to tell me that what I was experiencing was not normal. I remember she would laugh and say *"Abena it will pass just take it easy."* I was pregnant alright, but I was sick. My utmost desire was to be a Mum and here I was on that road but, I was sick.

Words of Encouragement

This is a point where it is very easy to begin questioning everything. Worry and fear may hit you and all the while you're just trying to understand what your body is doing. Remember motherhood is still the greatest honour and blessing despite how you are feeling. So far, you may be finding it challenging to maintain that thought and you may be wondering '*why me?*' This is understandable. The most important thing is that you don't keep everything bottled up inside. Speak to your midwife, partner or a friend and be encouraged.

This is a feeling that many of us have and it is not often understood by those who may have never seen such a condition, but your midwife/doctor has. For them to understand what you are experiencing you will need to tell them and to do that you will need to monitor what is happening to you. This includes keeping track of when you feel a change of mood. I must stress that sharing your anxiety and feelings with a health professional does not mean your baby will be taken away nor does it mean that you are an unfit Mum.

Often we fear to gain help within the Black, Asian and Minority Ethnic (BAME) communities due to stigma and potential future backlash or negative treatment once we share our true feelings. In addition to this black women specifically are often deemed as strong and are expected to take a lot. I must stress to you in childbearing there is no place for discrimination or in any healthcare for that matter. Despite my views on healthcare, BAME women are often treated differently when receiving care during antenatal and postnatal care. Therefore, I would encourage you to stand up for yourself. You know your body and you know what you feel. The moment you sit in front of a healthcare professional they are there to serve you and your baby - always try to remember that!

Below are a few steps you can take to prepare before attending antenatal care appointments:

- **Take someone with you for support**. It can get emotional when trying to express and describe what you have been going through in the early stages of pregnancy. This can bring up a whole load of emotions which may be difficult to keep under control; despite this it is still important to use this opportunity to share your feelings. Having someone there can enable you to stay focussed and also the person can advocate on your behalf if you are unable to. If you come into contact with a healthcare professional who is not listening to your concerns having someone there can provide the support you need to remain calm and articulate yourself, as the last thing you want is someone throwing the typical response for assertive BAME women of '*you are aggressive*'.

- **Take your notes along.** You may not have been keeping a log of your entire pregnancy experience but, you must have a rough summary of what has been happening whenever you attend appointments. Your notes should include how often you experience nausea and vomiting per day? When nausea and vomiting started? How often you eat and drink - specifically how much fluids you are getting? This can help the healthcare professional gain an understanding of your condition. It is unlikely that you will remember everything, and you certainly won't be able to demonstrate the full extent of your condition in a twenty-minute appointment, so your notes will come in handy.

- **Go in positive.** Be rest assured that at least now help is on its way. It's very easy to attend appointments already fed up which of course can be because of past experiences or our own negative thoughts on how we expect to be treated. If I am honest when it comes to this, I encourage you not to be in your way or become your barrier to getting what you need.

Remember that your feelings and questions about how you are feeling do not imply that you are ungrateful or don't understand the blessing of being pregnant. Nor does it mean that you do not deserve to be pregnant. Acknowledge how you feel and find methods that help you to push through and to endure the trials that sickness in pregnancy can bring.

Our culture/traditions encourage us to keep the pregnancy a secret for three months however, this may be near impossible depending on who you live with, the places you go and how sick you are. You haven't failed and you are suffering from a pregnancy-related sickness - hyperemesis gravidarum (HG).

A letter from my sister.

Dear Reader,

As you can imagine the news that there would be a new addition to the family filled me with complete joy. I would say that our family tree spans across a vast scope and a variety of countries. I already had 9 nephews, and even though I love them dearly, any chance of potentially gaining a niece was monumental. So, when my sister announced her pregnancy I couldn't wait for the arrival. However, the feeling of euphoria quickly diminished when I witnessed the effects that the pregnancy had on her. I expected her to suffer from morning sickness, but I quickly discovered that nausea and vomiting could happen at any point during the day, despite its name. I noticed that my sister seemed to always be experiencing nausea and sickness. This affected her energy levels and overall mood. It was obvious that she was happy about the pregnancy and that she couldn't wait to experience motherhood but, she could barely muster up a smile.

In the African culture, women seem to have developed the mindset of enduring everything without complaining even if you feel like you've been hit by a freight train. This meant that some relatives found it very difficult to accept that perhaps the rate in which my sister was losing fluids was down to a condition which could be dangerous. It wasn't until she was admitted to hospital and put on a drip that people realised the severity of HG. The lack of energy meant that fulfilling her everyday responsibilities became very tough and we had to provide support where we could. Unfortunately, her visits to the hospital were not a one-off and emptying her sick bucket became the norm. It was extremely challenging to watch not to mention off-putting. I certainly felt that I wouldn't want to have children if that's what it entailed. I remember feeling confused by the fact that her symptoms did not ease up even after the three-month mark. This led me to want to find out more and share my new-found knowledge.

Yours sincerely,

R. Nketia

2

THE DIAGNOSIS

Sitting in the doctor's office saying *"I keep being sick"* sounded like the most ridiculous statement ever.

"Of course you are being sick, you are pregnant. Pregnant women usually are sick." With tears in my eyes, I responded: *"But doctor I can't eat and I am continuously sick."*

"Okay but it will stop at three months." the doctor said. I took a deep breath and said: *"But doctor…. ok"*.

You see, I knew something was wrong, but I had never been in this scenario before. What does pregnancy feel like? Do all pregnant women get sick? I remember thinking about my friends who didn't, but hey the Doctor said it's normal so it must be normal… right? Trying to not be a burden I did as I was told and flowed with the pregnancy norms as listed in all the books and on all the apps. Until it went too far.

I had been experiencing so much nausea and vomiting that I had to move in with my parents as I was unable to hold anything down including water. The accident and emergency (A&E) department at the hospital was not where I wanted to be, but I was running out of options. I was eleven weeks pregnant and fed up with all the very unhelpful statements about how much I was vomiting and what I could do to stop it. Although I was given some anti-emetic tablets I had not taken them as prescribed because I was worried about taking medication while pregnant. I had no diagnosis of why I was so sick other than it being the usual pregnancy NVP. My baby bump looked five months and I could feel my anxieties growing. I had gotten so bad that I had no choice but to attend my local A&E for medical help. My sister took me in and as I stood at the desk to confirm my name my sister attempted to explain why I was there. As she spoke, I could feel myself becoming dizzy and then it happened. I fainted at the desk with my younger sister attempting to catch me. The lady behind the desk was so surprised she jumped up to look over at me in a heap on the floor. Extra staff were called, and I was rushed through and put in a cubicle on a bed.

After fainting, the doctor took some tests and the results highlighted my concerns to the A&E staff. I demonstrated that I truly was vomiting loads and as a result, there were ketones in my urine test. I was admitted to the ward, prescribed antiemetic medication, fluids and left to recover in my cubicle. Staff were so friendly and kind, but fear had overcome me as I watched three days pass by me.

During my hospital stay, there was a lady opposite me who didn't make eye contact with me and had her curtain closed the majority of the time. I concluded that I was either too friendly or I wasn't that sick. After all, everyone else didn't seem like they wanted to speak to me. It all made sense when the nurse explained that this ward had women who had varying pregnancy-related issues namely miscarriages, ectopic pregnancies and HG. During the medication round, the lady who was opposite finally locked eyes with me. It was literally like a movie. I seized the moment and greeted her, *"How are you feeling?"* I wanted to say, *'what are you in for?'* but that would have probably made her never speak to me again. She quietly said *"Hyperemesis!"* I stared at her puzzled.

That very day the consultant did a ward round and diagnosed me with HG. He let me know that this is not going to be easy and as I haven't stopped vomiting all the management methods they had tried hadn't worked. This meant that the next stage was for me to be given steroids. My emotions were mixed from confusion to relief that there was finally a reason behind why I was being sick. I continuously asked the lady opposite questions about HG as she was on her second child and, it seemed like her husband understood what was happening. I didn't expect her to be so real with me and share her deepest darkest fears. She managed to somehow empower me; I mean she was in a worse condition than me... right?

Later on, I shared the doctor's diagnosis with my Mum. It felt good to say, *"Mum they know what's causing it!"* Finally, there was a reason why I was vomiting. It wasn't the same condition as Grandma's friend's daughter, in Old Tafo town in Ghana, who was sick in 1986. It also hit me that I had a condition we had never heard of before. No one in my family had experienced this, and no one knew what this HG thing was. Moreover, I didn't know what this HG thing was. I was learning about my diagnosis daily, educating myself through HG groups, online and in books.

Then one day the doctors did their usual ward round and told the lady opposite that she had to improve, otherwise, her life was at risk. I looked on, listening through the cubicle curtain which offered little privacy. My eyes were filled with tears and my mind wondered, '*could having a baby be this difficult?*'

Words of Encouragement

By now you would know that HG is extreme, persistent nausea and vomiting during pregnancy. Getting a diagnosis of HG offers you the opportunity to:

- **Have an explanation for yourself.** Although it doesn't take away the sickness you can at least be rest assured that there is a reason why your body is behaving in this way.

- **You finally have something to say to others.** Yes, this is certainly not the time to be worrying about others but, the reality is your loved ones will want to offer you advice and support. Having a diagnosis is enough to zip a few mouths and send them off to do research. There may, however, be some people who will still feel compelled to share unwanted advice. A tip would be to send family and friends links to HG information sites. This will educate them on your recent diagnosis and hopefully reduce the talking.

- A diagnosis of HG offers you the chance to get the right support from maternity staff and receive the appropriate treatment. It also takes away the time and needs to prove that you were not just experiencing '*morning sickness.*'

At this point, I must stress to you that this is not your fault. You are not broken as I often told myself. Your body just handles pregnancy differently. According to the National Health Service (NHS) in the UK, it is not yet known why women suffer from HG nor is there a cure.[5] So, if you have HG you will have to come to terms with the fact that you will be in a state of what I called management. Once you accept this, it may not necessarily be easier, but things will start to look a lot clearer. You, with support from the health professionals, family and friends, will be required to manage! Day by day you will need to ride the wave of your pregnancy by:

---

[5]NHS Choices (2019). *Severe vomiting in pregnancy - Your pregnancy and baby guide.* [online] Available at: https://www.nhs.uk/conditions/pregnancy-and-baby/severe-vomiting-in-pregnancy-hyperemesis-gravidarum/

- Eating and drinking little and often (as best as you can);
- Resting;
- Taking the medication prescribed by your doctor; and
- Getting medical help at any point and every point you feel you need it.

Before we move on from this chapter I must home in on point four 'get medical help'. You know your body and while you may not know what being pregnant feels like you know if your body isn't feeling right. You know if you feel pain and you know if you are not coping emotionally. You also know if your intuition is speaking to you. No one will be fed up with you and if they are then quite frankly you don't want to be around them at this time. This includes in the hospital. You can be honest and say I don't think you are listening to me or I am concerned about XYZ. Where possible position a loved one to advocate for you during your pregnancy, this HG journey is a long one and while you may have done everything yourself in the past this season will teach you about needing and taking the help.

The pregnancy and hospital admission described in this chapter resulted in a miscarriage the day after I was discharged; despite me expressing that I was experiencing some pains before leaving the hospital that day. While I will never know why my baby became an angel after I had fought such a good fight, I feel it is important I share this, not to scare you but to reiterate that you need to listen to your body and force those caring for you to listen too.

3

ACCEPTANCE & MEDICATION

I was fortunate to have a Ghanaian midwife who not only understood HG but also understood my culture as my parents are also from Ghana. She was empathetic as she was aware that many people around me wouldn't know how to handle this HG thing. She prepared me for the possible responses to my diagnosis and encouraged me to stay focused. She challenged me not to take things personally, particularly other people's ignorance of the condition, unwanted advice and/or comparisons. Every appointment she gave me the space to talk about the ridiculousness of some of the comments I had received. We would laugh and she would offer me reassurance that I am doing ok whilst remaining respectful to the culture and traditions we shared. These fifteen minutes with my midwife empowered me so much as often between appointments; I had been admitted at least once. Her support and undivided attention meant a lot to me as she would also explore what had happened when I was admitted. The issue was when I left the appointment I felt like I was leaving people that understood me, so I often fell off confidence-wise.

As I was allergic to Cyclizine which is an antiemetic drug, I had been prescribed three other drugs to manage and control my nausea and vomiting. Metoclopramide, Polchloperizine and Ondansetron were my saviours at home and intravenous fluids when I was in the hospital. Despite all of these medical aids, I still kept vomiting. My midwife would constantly tell me to *"Take the meds on time and don't wait to get sick first."* This gave me so much confidence in my ability to take control of my HG as best I could. But, if I am honest as I sat in front of my loved ones (they truly love me), I often found myself thinking that they might be judging me. The question, *'how could a pregnant woman be taking so much medication?'* always played constantly in my head. This question had been asked in the past, and while no one was saying it to me now. After all they had watched me suffer so much and, all they desired was a healthy Mum and baby so there was nothing left for them to say or judge.

So what was stopping me from following the doctor's orders? Why would I miss doses or test myself and say, 'let's see if you can manage today'? The truth is denial along with a desire to be a *'normal'* pregnant woman. I desired and longed to go day to day without relying on medicines or thinking will I end up admitted today. By this point, I needed to get out of my way already and accept my reality. I had HG!

On the days I could wake up and get out of the house my medicines were safely tucked in the side part of my bag. I remember on one occasion as we left the house to go visit a friend Hubby looked back and asked, "*Have you got your medicine?*" I remember nodding and continuing to the car thinking he is only asking because he knows without it our fun will be cut short with my sickness. Knowing this became part of my journey to my acceptance phase and I was always prepared by packing my medicine, spare underwear and a bag to be sick in. This was life for the foreseeable future.

There was lots of information online about the individual medications I was taking; however, I did not venture to unravel these. I cast my mind back to the lady opposite my bed in the hospital and I was reminded that the doctor said her health was at risk. If you, the mother, are at risk then what about the baby? I, therefore, had no choice but to make decisions about my health which in turn will be of benefit to my unborn child.

Words of Encouragement

Here I am again reminding you that accepting your diagnosis doesn't mean you lack faith or you're not positive. It gives you the chance to at least give yourself a fighting chance of getting on top of and through this condition. Don't be like me; stop getting in your own way.

Let me put it in a scenario for you: if an elderly lady told you she needed help to walk but all she required from you each day was to put her walking stick next to her bed would you not do it? Not accepting and taking your medicine is like knowing you need a walking stick and putting it so far away that you are unable to ever get it. Every day you wake up and try to walk without it and then you fall (every day) hurting yourself. Your fall sends you right back to the beginning of your recovery because you are now injured. Just imagine!

Listen to your body.

I plead with you if you have been diagnosed with HG accept and prepare to fight through the journey. I am a firm believer in applying faith and wisdom in every situation. I was still vomiting when I took my medicine on some days and it was only my faith that was holding me up to a positive future. I knew that carrying this baby and staying healthy was a blessing. So remember your blessing. Remember your why. Accept how you feel. Apply wisdom and faith to deal with all of the above.

A letter from my Mum.

Dear Reader,

I knew that some women vomit throughout their pregnancy and that sometimes the vomiting can be triggered by even just a smell. Yet, I had never met a woman who was admitted due to excessive vomiting until it happened to my daughter. As far as I was aware pregnant women can only take folic acid (vitamins) daily and paracetamol once in a while, so seeing my daughter take lots of medication concerned me. I worried about the side effects that the medication may have on her and the baby. I empathised with my daughter, and so did her cousins. To help we often encouraged her and offered support even though we were concerned.

As a mother with a daughter with HG I learnt that it was important to listen to her concerns and encourage her to drink and eat little and often. No matter how much you know about the condition or your traditions, it is important to not add to her negative feelings but try to offer non-judgemental advice. Comparing her to other people because you have never experienced this before doesn't help and she will need to know that you understand her. I would urge you to stay focused on supporting and encouraging her through the difficult times.

Yours sincerely,

R. Owusu-Sekyere

4

WANTING TO GIVE UP!

Having lost a baby giving up wasn't an option. I had made a pact with God that if he gave me another chance at this motherhood stuff I would not give up. I might moan but, I won't give up. Several women are unable to continue their pregnancies to the end for several reasons. It is documented by The British Pregnancy Advisory Service (BPAS) that approximately 10% of women with HG terminate their pregnancy.[6] Having experienced HG it became a lot clearer why a lot of mothers make this decision. That being said, despite my decision not to terminate any of my pregnancies I want to reflect on a week in my third pregnancy.

Standing at the top of the stairs I wondered what would happen if I fell. Would the HG stop? Hubby was going out and by this time in my pregnancy, we had developed a system that I wouldn't be left alone. He dropped me off to my cousin's house and they were ever so welcoming but, I still felt like such a burden to them, my husband and my one-year-old daughter at the time. I had been vomiting all day which was now my new normal but on this particular occasion, I just could not shift the feeling of being a burden. My mind wandered to places it really shouldn't have and I thought if I fell down the stairs maybe I would shock myself into stopping the vomiting. But then I thought I could fall, break a limb, be admitted to hospital due to my broken limb and still be vomiting. Then I realised vomiting without broken limbs was far better than trying to manage broken limbs and HG together. Instead, I kissed my husband goodbye (on the cheek of course because HG doesn't make you feel worthy to kiss anything but, your mouthwash and toothbrush). By way of managing the overwhelming feelings of sadness I was having, I resorted to crying. I lay on the sofa in my cousin's house and cried, slept, cried and cried some more. This was one of the most emotional days I have ever experienced but also a very difficult day for those around me just watching on.

---

[6] www.bpas.org. (n.d.). | *BPAS*. [online] Available at: https://www.bpas.org/about-our-charity/press-office/press-releases/better-support-needed-for-women-with-severe-pregna/

There were so many things that triggered me that day and one thing for sure it was a day of acceptance for my situation. I had to accept that I had gone over the twelve-week mark which is often when HG stops and therefore, I was guessing this HG was here for the long haul. Going by my previous pregnancy I realised that I could potentially only stop vomiting one minute after my labour. All the possibilities of being in the percentage of those who don't get HG more than once, twice or even three times had gone out of the window. I was tired. I had to re-explain my condition to people who I had recently met, and I was just fed up.

To cope with my diagnosis, I had to take each day as it came and apply tools from my faith such as praying, reading and praying some more. I would tell myself to ignore them but, in reality, I would let people's views infiltrate what I felt in my situation. I will say a contributing factor to the negative effects on my mental health during my HG pregnancies is that people often had things to say. I would constantly be told, "Lick this, touch that, sniff this, eat this and my sister's friend did this and that." Sigh. It became exhausting trying to perform like a circus animal to do all the things I was being told to try. Although now I know they didn't mean any harm, at the time I was exhausted from trying to prove to people that I had tried everything they had said and more. As a result, it led me to feel like I had failed them.

Picture the scene, lying down and being asked over and over again, *'Rachael what should we give you to eat?'* If you have HG you will know that this is the most impossible question to answer, and if you were able to answer you probably no longer want it by the time you have finished saying it. On one occasion my cousin was concerned that I hadn't eaten anything at all. After I finally answered her question, and requested a cheese sandwich, my cousin rushed to make it and served me. My cousin is older than me so sending her here and there isn't something I would do confidently so, imagine how I felt when I sat up and ate some of this sandwich made with so much love, I suddenly felt like the world began spinning around. Then it came, I was sick. My cousin looked at me with the remainder of the sandwich and simply said *"oh."*

Words of Encouragement

Your mental health and well-being are paramount. HG can have an impact on you in a way you may not expect. Many women express that they are unable to complete their daily activities and all areas of living are affected while they suffer from HG. Being bedridden for the majority of the pregnancy is not the way NVP affects many women who experience *'morning sickness.'* While the physical effects may be obvious there is a major impact psychologically which may show in the form of anxiety and PTSD. You may feel isolation which if you are not used to being alone can feel very lonely and depressing.

If you have this book you have already made a step towards trying to help yourself manage or understand HG (insert me clapping for you). I can't tell you that it will be easy, but I can tell you will overcome it (even if it is at 39 weeks as the baby comes out.) You will overcome it!

Thinking about falling downstairs was not a good thought to have and I needed to have someone to be able to share such feelings with, as wild as they seemed. HG has a massive impact on you, physically and mentally so support is needed. Nothing you say is wrong and nothing you feel is wrong. You will need an outlet to talk so seek support from HG support sites that have volunteers who can listen and encourage you on this journey. Speak to your midwife about your thoughts and feelings as perinatal mental health is something that many people do not know about. Often all we know or hear about is postnatal depression, however, according to Mind.org.uk feeling depressed while pregnant affects one in five women.

I must stress that if you feel you are in a position where you're not being heard by the professionals you have notified of your feelings then it is very important that you stand up for yourself and seek help elsewhere. Putting it plainly if your midwife is not listening to you then tell someone else. Likewise if your doctor is not listening then tell someone else and keep talking until someone hears you.

I would encourage you to use a journal to capture your feelings and thoughts. This will act as a log which will help you to have a place to reflect on how far you have come. Every single day that you make it through, try to find a gratitude point to log in your journal to lift your spirits. It enables you to seek out positives in each day even on the days that may seem like the worst day of the pregnancy yet. Please know that you are blessed, and you will overcome it. Every day is an achievement, celebrate this and celebrate yourself. Tell yourself well done you made it through today.

As I said I can't tell you it's going to be easy but, I can tell you that you will get through this.

A letter from a friend.

Dear Reader,

So if anyone had asked me what HG was, I would not have had a clue! Despite being a mother of three myself all three of my pregnancies physically had been relatively easy, so when Rachael told me what she was going through I was completely clueless.

At first I did think it was just a case of extreme morning sickness and tried my best to offer the typical remedies, ginger biscuits, eating slowly etc. but I soon came to realise this was not just a case of extreme morning sickness.

I can't remember the date; I just remember calling her and thinking "No" this chick ain't right! So I quickly went to go and see what was going on!

Firstly I was just shocked that my friend who was so excited at having a baby looked so ill! Everyone knows in pregnancy you expect to gain weight, so why had my friend lost weight? Not only that but I heard the retching from the front door. I was just so shocked. Simple water to help her stay hydrated came flooding back out within seconds. I felt so helpless as there was nothing I could say or do to really comfort her.

The most frustrating thing was hearing about her going to the doctors several times and nothing being done to help her. It was like they just were not listening and that she was exaggerating her condition but how? You expect pregnant women to be glowing and healthy, bringing new life but my friend looked sick. She could barely put one foot in front of the other on the worst days. Every movement equalled throwing up!

I felt so sorry for her and guilty for my own smooth sailing pregnancies. I also felt guilty because I also didn't initially believe it could be as bad as she said. Another frustrating part was the lack of empathy that I think family members had for her. I guess sometimes it is hard to empathise with someone when you have not been there or experienced their situation, but the older generation also have a tendency to tell you to endure situations or be strong and get on with it without knowing the damage that not actually addressing the problem has on the person. So this was also an added pressure that I felt sorry that my friend had to endure.

Eventually after numerous doctor appointments and hospital visits Rachael was diagnosed with hyperemesis and I think the high profile of the Duchess of Cambridge also assisted in the condition bringing more prominence and a diagnosis being made. However just because a diagnosis was made it didn't mean that the medication worked. Being told that she had been admitted into hospital to be put on a drip more than once broke my heart. I just felt it just wasn't fair. How can you pray for something and do all the right things to prepare yourself for it and then when it finally happens your body basically rejects it?

Something that my friend had was strength to fight, she fought all the way until she gave birth. I want to encourage you to do the same. I would urge you to protect your mental health as best as you can by blocking out negativity and seeking help from people that are willing to listen.

Yours sincerely,
Y. Fofah

5

WORKING WITH HG

I was never one to consider the sick leave policy in great detail because I had never had an illness that would force me to think deeply about my job security. I had a knee operation many years before becoming pregnant and even then, work was very understanding, and the sick leave policy was fair. I knew the basics – if you become sick while pregnant it is a non-performance management issue and that pregnancy is a protected characteristic. This means that it is seen differently when implementing policies such as sickness monitoring. Apart from my general knowledge I had not looked into it.

With my first pregnancy, my symptoms came over me in the middle of my work car park. I was having a rough morning and had exchange students from France staying at my house. It was their last day, so I was dropping them to their pick up point and then making my way to work. I was on time and not stressed as my exchange students were 15-year-old boys, so they sorted themselves out and got in the car. I pulled up at work and my colleague said I had changed colour. Bearing in mind, I am black, and she too was a black woman so I knew that she understood the fact that brown skin may not show changes in the way it would in lighter skin tones. My colleague wouldn't allow me to enter the building as she was so concerned. I remember her insisting that I should not work that day. I felt like my world was spinning and my body was loading up for a serious outburst of vomiting. My eyes watered as I tried to hold my spinning head together.

I worked in education, so it is very common for sicknesses to be going around, so of course, my colleague and I put it down to me contracting a bug and I went home. That day I vomited several times as colleagues checked in and offered to drop things to my house. I genuinely felt love. I had been working there before I got married so everyone had been on the journey with me. I had a real family which included my 'work Mums and uncles.' When I found out I was pregnant it was fantastic news and all the staff celebrated with me. I worked as best I could until I found myself off sick again, and again and then for a long period.

Fast forward a few weeks and I was still not getting better and ended up being off work for many months. This was not cool. I had to seek help from a doctor as I realised that this wasn't going to be an easy ride. I had barely gotten to grips with my condition let alone those around me. My employer was very concerned but knew my work ethic, and therefore there was no distrust in what I was saying regarding how I was feeling. I was free to be honest and expressed that the way that I was feeling was shocking me as much as it was shocking them. My manager was supportive throughout the journey and encouraged me to seek medical help with my condition. It was clear that it was quite an unpleasant experience, and I appreciate that this kind of support is not the case for many HG sufferers.

By my second pregnancy I had a routine; I would wake up, have a cup of tea, take some medication and allow that all to sink in. Despite the medication I would usually still vomit. Once I had vomited I would then prepare myself for work, get ready and leave but, I knew that when I got in the car I would probably be sick again. To prepare for this I carried a sick bag in the car. It would usually be only a short distance away from my house that I would find myself vomiting again. I would have to pull over and get out of the car with my bag and vomit. This impacted my journey to work so I often had to leave earlier than planned to accommodate for the possibility of feeling unwell enroute. I also had to ensure that I carried a spare set of clothes especially, spare underwear, for moments when I had been violently sick and potentially wet myself or vomited on my clothes. Yes, it was that serious. Once this was all done I would continue my journey to work and get through the day until about lunchtime when I would tend to vomit straight after eating. There was a room at my work where you could go and rest during your break, I would frequent there to lie down and recoup. I was often seen rushing in and out of the lunch hall so that I had enough time to go and lie down in that room and pull myself together ready for the afternoon.

On some days this routine didn't work, and I would have to turn back on my way to work or leave work early due to uncontrollable vomiting at work. It was absolutely devastating for me as I would continuously vomit and still try to do my job. A job that required me to use my full capacity, and often stand in front of a class of students feeling nauseous. It was very challenging knowing that they needed me to deliver the lesson so that they could gain the knowledge.

I recall one occasion when I arrived at work and I sat at my desk and ate a sausage. The first thing my friend who sat next to me said was "Oh dear, no wonder you'll be sick you're eating a greasy sausage at nine in the morning!" What she didn't know was that I hadn't eaten for most of the weekend. I was worried about getting dehydrated and I was genuinely hungry. I saw the sausage and I fancied it and even if I got to lick or just to taste a little bit of it I would have been happy. What she said made me feel embarrassed and anxious, almost as if I had chosen to make myself sick. On a normal day, I eat sausages and to be fair sausages had not made it into my relegated list of foods, so it was something I could eat without vomiting. Besides who gave her the right to comment on what I ate and when I can eat? Did she know what I had been through over the weekend? Did she know how much I needed food to stay well? Did she know that it was a struggle for me to get into work that morning? Sigh. I would then think 'Did she mean any harm?' The fact is the answer to all of the questions is no, she didn't. She didn't know much about my condition and she didn't take the time to. This was not because she didn't want to but, she was probably fed up of me being sick next to her. She didn't consider how fed up I may have been too.

As she sat next to me, I felt like I had to eat that sausage in secret. Later that day I did vomit but whether that had anything to do with my sausage I will never know nor would my colleague. I'm sure she sat there feeling like saying, "I told you so". Unbeknown to my colleague this little conversation controlled what I ate in the office due to fear of judgement and comments that would make me feel like I had caused my HG. I must say that this colleague was a friend and we got along really well; she meant no harm, but she caused great harm. This made me realise that I needed to put up some boundaries around my health and my condition. Allowing anyone to comment and say what they think at any given time on what I ate was detrimental because it could set me back from eating as well as I could for the day.

Words of Encouragement

Remember how difficult it is to get your family to understand the condition? This is the same difficulty you may have in your place of work. HG is unknown to many therefore many will lack the knowledge and understanding of the condition and the way that it affects you. They do not know what you are experiencing and the severity of it. While you are in the thick of feeling unwell it may not be your priority to try and justify your condition to anybody so you must use some tools such as online information to support you. Send the information over to your employer/colleagues for them to understand what your condition is. Be sure to seek out occupational health support for them to also help you with explaining your condition to your employer that way you have their backing.

I wish I could tell you that all employers will believe that you have HG and you are suffering but, unfortunately not all will understand or know anything about it. You may be the first person that they have ever come into contact with HG and that's not your fault nor your problem. All you can do is give them the information they need so that they know about you and your condition.

If you are bedridden with HG it is easy to want to block out the whole world but try to ensure that you follow all of your organisation's policies and procedures. This will ensure unnecessary contact and pressure is not placed on you. For example, if your employer has not received a sick note from you they will not know that you are sick. This may sound like common sense and you may feel so rough that this is not a priority but notifying your employer of your sickness and absence will, in turn, end up reducing your stress of them looking for you. It will also help you maintain your responsibilities and relationship with your employer.

If at any point you feel that you are unable to make those contacts then assign this to a family member or a friend. They can ensure that your sick notes are posted and that you've responded to emails regarding your return to work. Just make sure that this is someone you can trust to do it.

Unfortunately, you will need to set yourself a very clear routine which accommodates and allows for your potential vomiting spouts. If you feel you can still work then you need to:

- Allow additional time in your movement plans to be able to accommodate for feelings of nausea or vomiting. Waking up earlier, taking pauses in your preparation time and planning your route will give you the much-needed stop off points if you need to be sick.

- Make sure you always have a spare set of clothes and cleaning products in your car/bag in case you vomit and need to clean up after yourself. I must stress that you always pack a spare set of underwear because the vomiting can be so violent you may want to change.

- Pack some snacks in your car/bag and keep it in a place where you can reach it. The worst thing is getting stuck in traffic or being on public transport with no snacks or water.

- Make sure that when you do come home from work you rest to recuperate and be ready for the next day. This is the time where you may not be able to work at home in the evenings unless you feel that's the time when you feel better than you do in the day.

- Set boundaries at work, you are with your colleagues more than you are even with your family depending on how many hours you work; it is very easy for people to begin to tell you what to do and when. While you may have really good relationships with these people when you are pregnant with HG some of their comments will potentially irritate you. You should set boundaries as there are certain things that you just don't want to hear. If you have a good relationship with your colleagues then let them know that you are suffering from HG. You can signpost them to research or articles about HG but, you do not have to sit and explain yourself every time you attempt to eat a meal or are vomiting.

- Do not allow people who do not understand your situation to feel brave and close enough to comment on it. It will add undue stress to the situation. Now I'm not saying don't take advice or speak to a friend but, just be mindful that as you spend so much time at work you don't want to open up conversations that will have a negative impact on your mental health.

If you feel that your condition and your symptoms are too much then stay home! Going to work under any type of pressure to prove something to somebody or to prevent activation of sickness monitoring is not necessary. You are a pregnant woman with HG therefore, you are protected and covered by the laws of the land. It is not a requirement for you to attend work while sick, it is a requirement for you to attend work and do your best when you can function. Therefore, do not allow anyone to pressure you into working when you feel unwell as your health and the baby's health is paramount. Again, I know it may sound silly that this is part of my words of encouragement but, when you are vulnerable, under pressure and being told that what you have is just pregnancy sickness, you will find yourself trying to force yourself to do things that you just can't. You may find working at full capacity in the way you used to impossible due to HG and that's ok.

6

FUNCTIONS AND OUTINGS

Being the life and soul of the family, functions are often planned by me, attended by me, and the fun that we have is usually activated by me. Being aware of this made the fact that I was not able to go out or be present at a family function quite hard to deal with. Having to explain to people why I could not come and could not do things, especially when I wanted to go also made it difficult.

HG and its unpredictability requires the acceptance and acknowledgement that you may become limited in terms of being able to go out when you want to go out. This doesn't mean that you won't struggle with the idea, and I can truly testify that it is a struggle. I remember it being my God-Daughter's birthday and I wanted to be there packing party bags, dressing tables and generally coordinating the whole event. I have always been quite an active person in the lives of all the children in my life, however, for this occasion; I had to take a complete step back because I was unwell due to HG. I exhausted every possible way that I could get involved from phone to WhatsApp but, the reality was I was limited. The good thing was my God-Daughter's Mum worked in the profession that exposed her to several women with HG, so she knew and understood the limitations. This was significantly helpful when it came to dealing with the feelings that I had about not being able to be involved or be there. I know I keep banging on about acceptance but, when I accepted that I was unable to do certain things I remained calm and managed to show my face at my God-Daughter's party. Now to some, you may be thinking why you didn't just stay at home but, for me, it was so important for me to be there. Many other times I had to sit it out, stay at home and watch functions through videos that people sent through WhatsApp or conversations of the description of what was going on. This was as close as I was going to get.

In our culture funerals are a very big deal, often running over three days. On the second day (after a burial) we often celebrate life and Ghanaians dress up in the specified dress code colour, present money and dance to celebrate the life of the person who has passed on. I was unable to attend such events. Imagine being sad about being unable to attend a funeral.

Contributing to funeral costs is also significant within our culture as well as showing your support by attending the event. So whenever funerals came up, I was met with the possibility of having to explain to somebody who doesn't understand what HG is and attribute this as the reason why I was not present. After months of this, and especially during my last pregnancy my husband and I had to create a system that worked for us. On occasions, my husband would go and be present and represent both of us. This would again mean that I would have to stay at home or go to my cousin's house to be looked after while he was out of the house.

A time that has never left me is when Hubby went to an event that was live-streamed via Facebook. I logged on and watched everything that was going on whilst lying in bed as I was unable to sleep. I found myself listening to music, laughing at the MCs jokes and pretending that I was there as a way of coping with the fact that I couldn't go. For many going out isn't that important when you're growing a life but, not being able to go out because of something that my body was doing was a whole different thing. It's like when someone says don't lick your lips and somehow all of a sudden you needed to lick your lips. Similarly, the moment that the option of going out is taken away from you because of something debilitating and mentally exhausting the mind slips into a place of negativity.

The issue was not, just not being able to go to an event. It was also a challenge trying not to be sick while getting dressed and of course, having a limited choice of outfits because your bump is growing faster than your ability to do maternity shopping. Then there was the makeup, this required sitting or standing in front of the mirror for way longer than I could manage or wanted to. Taking a shower was also a lot of effort as the standing up was exhausting to the point that I often found myself wondering if it was worth it. To be fair most times it ended up in me being sick. The getting ready process just seemed extremely tedious and almost felt like I was rocking the boat unnecessarily as it often ended with me feeling worse. Sigh.

Alas, we continued to use the system of Hubby going to events that I couldn't go to and me only attending events that I could manage to go to. Even if this was for the whole pregnancy.

I nearly missed my friend's wedding; I've known this friend for many years, so I was desperate to go. The issue arose when the hospital asked me to come in on the morning of the wedding for them to monitor the baby, check for ketones and that everything was ok. I arrived at my appointment in a pink gown with a huge fascinator on my head and as expected every single person in the hospital turned their heads to look at me as if to say I was completely mad. I placed a thick TENA Lady pad in my underwear just in case I had a bout of vomiting that caused me to pee a little as I vomited. I didn't want to ruin my dress. I remember sitting in the doctor's room looking at the nurses and doctors with beady eyes in the hope that everything was ok for me to be able to go to the wedding. After urine samples and monitoring the baby's heart rate, I was finally told that I'm ok to go to the wedding but, I had to be careful, go home early and get some rest. So I went to the wedding even though I was late, and managed to see my friend get married. For me this felt like a step forward.

When I was pregnant with my daughter, I had a business that hosted baby showers so I knew what type of baby shower I wanted. I spent several days on my sick bed planning my ideal baby shower against the wishes of my family and friends who were trying to plan it for me. The only issue was I was still quite unwell and I didn't even know if I could still make it to the baby shower. I remember the makeup artist arriving just after I had vomited and I took my medication so that I could get through the makeup session. I didn't really care about what style she did as I knew it would be better than how I looked. Once she finished the makeup I put on a blush pink gown and I felt extra and looked amazing on the outside, but inside I was scared. I knew that if I vomited now I would ruin the whole event that so many people had worked hard to put together. Along with the medication my friends made me sit up whilst I slept for half an hour before the event to try and stop me from vomiting. Once all the guests arrived and the games were about to start they picked me up and took me to the hall. Whilst I looked glamorous and happy there was discrete monitoring going on to jump in, in case I needed to be sick. During the speeches, we all cried because we knew how hard this journey had been.

When I was pregnant with my son I had already started my business, which was a network for Mums, and I attempted to blog my motherhood journey, however, due to being unwell, it was inconsistent. I had seen several pictures and photoshoots online that I really wanted to do with my daughter and my bump, but I knew this would be difficult. There was the unpredictability of my health and the issue of finances, so I needed a photographer who would be able to understand that my HG could affect the photoshoot. Fortunately, I met a photographer called Iko-Ojo Mercy Haruna who had also suffered from HG herself, and she was also looking for someone who was pregnant to do a photoshoot with. Her own experience with HG enabled her to be patient with me during the photo shoot, which is something I am eternally grateful for. In appreciation for all her hard work and support, I wrote the following email to her:

Dear Mercy,

I am passionate about supporting fellow mamas and their business but truly went out of my comfort zone in several areas to just get to this shoot today. That said at every hurdle we overcame. The messages, planning and discussing all came together and it was over and beyond what I could have imagined.

When you have hyperemesis, pelvic girdle pain (PGP) and every other pregnancy symptom going you do not feel gorgeous, yummy mummy or even have a pregnancy glow. I have literally been existing in my skin and focusing on being an incubator. Hair combing, makeup and dressing up are the last thing on my mind around potty training and eating to stay alive. Today's shoot did more than capture the most amazing experience of carrying my second child and sharing that with my precious daughter. It did more than show my nice outfits and my matching accessories. It touched my heart. I cried because it reminded me that I am actually in those images. It is actually me! I am more than pregnancy pain, sickness and all the other life stresses one may be facing at any given time. I looked at the images and the comments you guys were making and I thought wow "I am actually alriiiiight init".

Yes, my back arches, and yes my child's cornrows weren't fresh, and yes my bump was lopsided at a point but, all of those things made me even more beautiful. It made what I am currently experiencing even more special. Thank you so much for this shoot. The healing strand that flows through each picture hugging a pregnant hormonal stressing mama is indescribable. May God truly bless you.

I may still look mash up until I give birth as the pregnancy enters the end-stage but, at least I have memories of the temporary suffering I went through for the beautiful privilege of being a second-time mama.
Love Rach.

Words of Encouragement

You see HG will create uncertainty and spontaneous changes in your plans and you realise that your events will not be like everyone else's. Be encouraged that it will pass even if that is after you have given birth; the main thing is this is not forever. There are a few things that you can do to help yourself cope:

1.   *Take away guilt.*

- Do not allow guilt to make you lose focus. You are doing the most amazing thing - carrying your precious baby. You may miss someone's special day or something you so much desired to attend but, honestly, this is not your fault or you being difficult. This is you looking after you and the baby.

- A way to lessen the feeling of guilt is to send a gift, message or card showing you were thinking of the person. You may find this makes you feel like you have not ignored the occasion.

- Although, this may result in the person giving you a response that is insensitive because of their lack of awareness of HG, have a conversation with the person hosting the event. Just make sure that you time this conversation wisely. Imagine trying to tell someone what you are going through while they are rushing around trying to sort out their biggest event. While they may have the utmost empathy towards your situation the truth is you may not receive that at the time you have chosen. Be warned.

- Send your spouse/friend on your behalf to represent you.

2.   *Prepare for a change of plan.*

- Things will take you longer or just generally become annoying to do. You will need an extra 10 minutes to put on shoes or even to vomit, so it is important to be prepared.

- Choose outfits in advance of an outing as this will save you time and frustration of trying things on.

- Always have a backup outfit. I appreciate this may not be possible if you are wearing the chosen cloth for the occasion which is also known as Aso Ebi. Where possible keep a strip of the fabric as a backup, that can be tied like a waistband (well under the boob band) if you get my gist.

- Put your outfit on last. Simple but effective. There is no point stressing out in your outfit.

3.   *Be realistic with your responsibilities.*

If you have to do things before an event or you already have a child, then it is important that where possible you ask for help. You haven't failed! You just need some help. One of the common mistakes we make as women is not asking for help, as well as us not being specific about the help we need. Expecting your partner, Mum or friend to just know what and how you want something done is setting yourself and them up to fail. Be clear and be honest. If you can get help, then say exactly what you need. Be patient though! The helper may not do it how you have done it for the past five years, but they are trying. You are not ungrateful if you don't like how things are being done, however, as with everything we must reflect and respond tactfully.

I will talk more on HG while raising other children further into the book but in terms of responsibility for children when going out again try to say exactly what you need. If you need to type a list on your phone to forward, then do so as this will help you and your helper to understand what you want. Be patient though! Again your helper may take time to get to grips with what your child needs and the way HG is set up, to be honest, you may be at the point of 'as long as the child comes out alive.' What they wear and how many sweets they eat becomes a secondary matter.

4.   *Don't offer your services.*

Coming from an African household not asking what you can do to assist is like a serious abomination. As in someone will quote and refer to you how they may have helped you in the past or your mother may suggest you call your cousin Ama to support her for her wedding. My dear Mama reading this book - FORGET IT! HG is unpredictable so unless you are through the worst of it and can bear it do not put yourself in a place of service. Yes, I said it! You cannot cook your famous Jollof for three hundred people, nor can you wrap six hundred favours. Most importantly do not take on what you cannot handle.

The worst thing you can do is let someone down at the last minute and then be riddled with guilt inside for ruining a part of their event. I appreciate that people may ask you to do things but, do what is best for you and use the simple word we were all so confident to say as children NO! You can explain and suggest sending the recipe for your special Jollof or signpost them to someone who can help them. HG can impact your mental health immensely and this condition can leave a long-lasting impact on you, so the last thing you need to add is the pressure of party Jollof.

A letter from my God-daughter's mum.

Dear Reader,

I have known Rachael since we were infants. She had always been very vocal from a young age that she wanted a large family. I was waiting for decades in anticipation, for the moment she announced she was going to be a mother. I was so elated when she did and as she began to experience, what at the time I deemed to be morning sickness, I drew from my journey as a form of encouragement. Reassuring her that it often subsided by the afternoon and by the end of the first trimester, it would most likely be all over. Except this didn't happen, the episodes become more frequent and increasingly ferocious.

Rachael and I often spoke most days and I would be on the other end of the line, as she wretched and tried to hold down any little she may have consumed. It took some time before I realised what was happening. I recalled a client I encountered as a student, who frequented the hospital with constant nausea and vomiting due to pregnancy, which required an inpatient stay and 24 hourly intravenous fluid infusions. It has also been 7 years but I have never forgotten her and the despair in her face, as she contemplated having a termination because she could no longer bear it. It was just agonising to watch, as she turned up to the hospital time after time, often with her three-year-old son, to find out that there was very little we could do. When I realised this was Rachael's fate, I felt helpless. I realised from both a personal and professional capacity, she was alone.

As the weeks passed, I was seeing less and less of the Rachael I had become accustomed to. She was vanishing before my eyes. The once exuberant and outgoing friend I knew, had become withdrawn and anxious about the most basic of tasks, barely mustering the strength to leave her bed in the morning; a combination of being up all night and weakness due to the continuous vomiting. The hardest part was watching her attempts to proceed as normal, compounded by her recent appointment at work, almost as if she was in denial. I often pleaded with her to call off sick but, she just wouldn't hear of it, she didn't want to let them down. Yet she was clearly in no condition to teach and spent most of the morning, including her commute, having to pull her car aside to vomit along the way to work. I didn't understand how she made it through, only to rise the subsequent morning and do it all again. It was evident mentally it was taking its toll on her and aside from our comfort calls, she didn't have much perinatal mental health team support to help her navigate the challenges she faced day-to-day. My empathy only went so far, she was ultimately alone and it was heart-wrenching to watch.

My natural instinct is to always try to fix things and/or offer suggestions according to my own experience and in situations like this, that approach is almost futile. This condition was anything but predictable and no matter how much I supported and assisted her to manage daily, she was in this alone. It was happening to her and ultimately there was very little I could practically do, but to pray. Faith is all I could cling onto and use to remind her that this trial will ultimately turn out to be a testimony. We don't always have to save the day, sometimes we simply just need to surrender and understand we don't have the answers to everything, and that's okay. It was emotionally a lot for us all, but I believe just being a friend and being there, is enough. It is the little things that matter.

Yours sincerely,

J. Apaloo

7

FINANCIAL ISSUES

Having children generally costs money so I had always been aware and prepared for the financial challenges that having a child would bring. What I wasn't prepared for was HG and whilst preparing for the upcoming income changes during maternity leave was a high priority the priorities changed dramatically from being prepared to staying alive, well and healthy.

Knowing I was going to have a baby meant I was set up for at least eight months preparation time which included pre-maternity leave money. I had planned it all out in a way that I would make the most of my pregnancy time to save more, reduce my monthly outgoings and be more frugal before the baby came. This seemed like a smart way to do things at the time until HG hit me. You see, what I hadn't planned for was long periods off sick, which happened in each pregnancy and affected my pay each time. On all three occasions of me having HG, I spent several days, weeks and even months off work at a time. Once my sick pay allowance finished, I was then paid a reduced amount following the organisation's policies. This left my plan shattered into pieces and I was not in a position where I could just force myself to work for the money due to how unwell I was. My bills had not reduced, and my financial forecast had not miraculously changed to accommodate HG. This in itself is stress I didn't need. Whilst I appreciated the fact that there was another income in the household I must be transparent in this reflection, and say the financial situation was not ok for several reasons. The sheer fact that I was the one carrying the baby and creating additional financial problems for the household was an awful feeling. This feeling was made worse with the fact that I had never been out of control of my finances. I knew what was coming in and what money was going out, when, to who and why. I felt responsible for rocking what was a stable financial boat and of course it wasn't my fault, but I still felt a way about it.

My eating habits created another financial impact on the household simply because if I got the taste for a particular thing then we needed to get it right then. I rarely ate because I wanted to or fancied a particular thing; I ate because I had to, and so when I did get the taste for something, we were all happy. My pregnancy palette was a little bit strange at times, requesting school dinner style meals and lobster or grilled salmon at random times of the day. After weeks of witnessing me not eat well the words *"Babe I fancy..."* became music to my Hubby's ears. He would rush out and grab it, but he wouldn't buy one or two he would buy loads of that one thing.

Straight after eating whatever it was, I was craving at the time I would vomit and not want any more of it, ever again. This method of grocery shopping became quite costly and before we knew it, we would have spent way over the budget for weekly shopping. My Hubby's way of responding to my cravings would result in as much as £30 worth of salmon in the fridge that I won't eat. This didn't help our bank balances nor my nausea, but as time went on, I realised it was deeper than just doing ad hoc shopping. Hubby had the bigger picture in mind, which was to give me everything I needed, especially food-wise to ensure I had taken something in and was not dehydrated. As a self-employed worker Hubby couldn't afford to take time off work to be with me in hospital, therefore he needed to support me in maintaining my health as a hospital admission would mean two incomes had been affected. As time went on, I had no choice but to be in the hospital and he didn't leave my side except on the odd occasions to work when he knew I had other family members around to visit.

Words of Encouragement

In 2020 Money Supermarkets stated the average cost was £79,176 to raise a boy and £108,884 for a girl and as the cost of living goes up so can the cost of having a family.[7]Finances and having children have always been an issue, and honestly, it takes a lot to be fully financially prepared for having children as there is always something changing or needed. However, you can plan and put in strategies to adapt if things do not go to plan.

HG may leave you without a salary and I cannot give you a magic theory as to how you will generate funds during this time, but here are some things to consider:

- **What help is available?** : Long periods of sickness often result in a pay drop to statutory sick pay - dependent on the organisation's set sick leave policy. Check with your employer, charities and government guidance to see what financial support is available to you during your long periods of sickness. For example, there are organisations in place for you to gain advice on managing your

---

[7] @moneysupermkt. (2019). *How Much Does It Cost To Raise A Child? | MoneySuperMarket.* [online] Available at: https://www.moneysupermarket.com/life-insurance/cost-of-raising-a-child/

outgoing payments when you have reduced or no salary. Don't be afraid to seek this information out nor to seek help; after all, asking a question is not a crime. Often, we feel that having a child is our choice and therefore, no one else's problem. However, if there are systems in place for us to get advice/support then we should. Remove the stigma around asking for help. This is the one time in your life you will need to get help in several ways.

- **Save:** Before you run out and buy loads of baby stuff just hold off for a minute. Acceptance of your current circumstances is about you acknowledging that your story is not like anyone else's. Don't run out and buy loads of bits for the baby just yet. Focus on managing and maintaining your financial situation now and have faith that tomorrow will be handled. Save what you can but do not allow the need to save to turn into anxiety. You may not meet your saving goals as you had planned prior to having HG but, you will have your baby and you will find a way to manage even if it's not your ideal way.

- **Make money:** As your baby grows in the womb you may find yourself nesting and this a fantastic time to get rid of stuff that you no longer need but, don't throw things away. Sell them on platforms that sell used and new goods. This will bring in money that you never had for things that you no longer need.

- **Go easy on yourself:** Finances have always been something we are encouraged to keep private within our culture. Debt and needing money is often hidden and can cause very negative feelings. So just imagine having HG and internalising negative feelings about your finances. HG is not the same as being reckless with money as a teen and ending up in debt for the rest of your life. HG is a debilitating condition that can cause you to be in a position where you are unable to make an income for some time. This is completely out of your control.

8

HG WHILE RAISING A CHILD

When I fell pregnant, it was not part of the plan at the time. My son came as a complete surprise, so I certainly hadn't prepared my mind for HG for the third time. A week before I found out that I was pregnant I began to feel pain in my bum but, I didn't think it was a symptom of pregnancy. I remember the pain started as I was walking around the shopping centre with friends, so I asked them if they were feeling tired of walking too. My friend insisted that we go to a drug store and buy a pregnancy test because she thought I was pregnant. I disagreed with her and explained that it couldn't be the case and that I wouldn't rush to a shop and take a pregnancy test in the middle of a shopping centre in the toilet. I was quite defensive, and I kept emphasising that I would know if I was pregnant.

As the days went on, I thought she might be right. Three days later, I found out I was pregnant when my daughter was off sick from nursery. I rushed to the doctor's to get her seen and found out that she had a common childhood illness. The illness meant that she had to stay off nursery for at least one week. On the way back home I bought a pregnancy test pack that came with three tests. I got home, put my daughter down to sleep upstairs, and noticed that I felt extremely tired, but I still wanted to have me time and watch a programme. I went to the toilet to take the test. As I put it on the side I noticed a second faint line and I was astonished. I walked away, ignored it and then I went back and looked at it again. I slowly crept downstairs, sat in silence on the sofa then, it hit me. I called my friend and I remember saying to her "*So your girl is about to be a Mum of two.*" Boy, oh, boy, were we in shock.

Incidentally, I had been feeling extreme tiredness and couldn't put my finger on what it was. With the flu and colds going around at the time I used it as an excuse, but it didn't make sense as I had been bleeding the month before which I automatically had put down to an irregular period. I remember that period was very unpleasant. I was looking after my daughter at the time and on top of that, I had to deal with this overwhelming feeling of nausea and my unexpected period. My Hubby took my daughter out that day and allowed me to sleep. I pulled myself together and felt able to step out for a bit. I couldn't stay out long though because I was bleeding heavily. The heavy period lasted for three days, after which I resumed a normal period cycle flow.

Reflecting on that day I immediately called the hospital and explained that I had just taken a pregnancy test and it came out positive, but I also had an irregular heavy period the month before. They asked me to come in straight away because of the bleeding I had. On arrival, I was fortunate to get an early scan to see what was happening. I felt so overwhelmed with emotion as you can imagine, I was having a first scan within hours of finding out that I was pregnant. I called my friend who rushed to meet me at the hospital so that she could hold my daughter. Whilst I was lying on the bed the doctor asked how I was, and I couldn't find the words to answer except laugh. I felt dumbstruck as I had gone from being tired and worried about my daughter to now potentially having two children and HG. As I lay there she explained that I may need to have an internal scan. During the scan, she told me that she could see the baby and that I looked about six weeks pregnant. I was so shocked that all I could do was stare at her. I'm not sure if she knew what to say and I certainly didn't know what to say. I took a deep breath and just said *"Wow! I'm pregnant."* I'd not met this doctor before, but she offered such reassurance and warmth. This encouraged me to think positively and leave that room happy. I wish I wrote down her name because I appreciated the support in that first moment of finding out I was pregnant.

I remember her asking, *"Did you want more children?"* and in response, I said, "Yes but, I am worried about HG." She instantly said *"You can do this! You are blessed and you will be ok."* All I can say is that God stepped in and gave me the confirmation I needed that everything was ok because I don't think I could have slept thinking the worst. I thought that the period I had may have been a miscarriage. As I walked out of the assessment, my friend stared at me as if to say *"Well…"* and I looked back at her like a child on her first day at school and said, *"Yep, I'm pregnant."*

It's awfully strange how as women we often try to protect everyone around us except for ourselves. Even though I had one of the most emotionally challenging days of my life at no point did I inform my husband. I was so concerned about getting his hopes up and then panicking him in light of the previous bleeding. I felt the need to protect him from what was happening, and I also think that I was doing it for myself too. I waited until he arrived home that evening, and when he arrived home, he was greeted by our daughter handing him a drawing on which I had written *'Mummy has a baby in her tummy'.* He looked at me as if I had lost the plot and looked around the room like someone was going to jump out and say that this was all a joke. I remember him looking at me and saying, *"Oh my goodness,"* and then he gave me a massive hug.

The next morning I woke up and it fully hit me that I was a pregnant woman and I would soon be a mother of two children under three. I quickly dealt with that, but the struggle was waking up and showing all the signs and symptoms of someone suffering from her HG. In less than 24-hours after discovering that I was pregnant, nausea hit me, and I immediately regretted knowing that I was pregnant after all. I started to wonder if I had just brought HG onto myself. I questioned whether this was all in my head. I had already begun to panic about how long this journey is going to be.

Now I had a young baby and a growing foetus and as time went on, I felt less and less able to do the things I needed to do or that I usually did. Waking up on time and getting my daughter ready all became a very slow process. We live so far away from my Mum that it meant that I just had to manage and to be fair she also had her own job. Hubby worked while I tried to continue as normal, but it began to show when my daughter's hairstyles didn't change weekly, and I could barely get the laundry done in time for nursery the next week. You would think it would be easier to call someone to come and help. Yet, I was quite selective of who I let in my space after an experience that left me feeling inadequate as a wife and mother. I got a call from a family member who happened to be in my area and asked if she could come by. I had been unwell and home alone with my daughter for two days, so I was excited to see another adult. Knowing that she was family I felt comfortable with her coming into my environment as it was. As she entered the house she commented on the laundry that I had folded but left in the basket on the dining table. She referred to the place as being messy, but it had taken everything in me to fold those clothes before she arrived. This put me off asking for help and having any more visitors unless my husband was present to fix or justify the state of the house.

Eventually, I was unable to work for quite some time and the only lifesaving thing that I had was the fact that my daughter went to nursery. I would drop her to nursery late usually because I had been vomiting in the morning and often would be sick during the drop-off. The nursery was so understanding, and you would often find me in their waiting area trying to pull myself together after finally managing to drop her off. I would sit outside the nursery for an hour or two either being sick or feeling extremely nauseous and unable to drive. Sometimes I would just sleep outside until I could eventually drive myself home and sleep for the rest of the day; so much so that one day I was fined as I had overslept.

As time went on my little princess who was not even two yet begun to realise Mummy wasn't well. She would bring me a makeshift bucket when we were home alone as soon as she heard me heave and would often ask "*Mummy okay?*"

Those thirty-eight weeks of pregnancy made her mature fast and I was so grateful that she was so confident verbally from such an early stage. I felt I could reason with her about what was happening to me and why I couldn't do anything. This scenario was not filled with lots of child-free days where I could focus on managing my HG, and for many of us, that will be the case. I did feel guilty on many occasions that this baby was looking after me more than I was looking after her. I must remind you she was only one year old. She comforted and cuddled me, which was so mature, yet she still snuck into my room at night sometimes.

As much as I love my child so much, she was a massive contributor to my sickness. Her morning nappy would send my whole existence into disarray. I would be overwhelmed with nausea and vomiting just to change her nappy. I became afraid to do it because I knew it would stop us from functioning for the day. So we had to find a solution. My husband would leave for work quite early, but it now became his responsibility to change her nappy before he left, so when she woke up even if I changed her again it wasn't too bad.

Her food options changed to what I could manage to smell whilst making it, and healthy snacks were a must. This was key for me because hospital admissions were the last thing I wanted. I needed to stay home for my baby therefore; I needed to manage the situation. Her outings were also majorly affected. Sometimes I felt able to go out but, when I wasn't family members would step in or Hubby would do the honours. Does she remember anything from that time? No, I thought it was the worst thing for her to have to experience, but she was only one at the time, now nearly five years old and she doesn't seem to remember. I show her videos of us with my bump but, it's all just a distant memory.

Words of Encouragement

I can't tell you that raising a child while suffering from HG is going to be easy. Honestly, it isn't, however, there are some things you could try to do to help you best manage:

- **Request help.** As mentioned above, be sure to ask for help and be specific when highlighting what you need. Often people feel like they don't want to step on your toes or offer help where it's not needed so reach out to your family and friends and be specific.

- **Plan and prepare.** Always plan your items when you are manoeuvring with your child. Prepare the bag and the clothes when you're feeling well enough to, so that you reduce the pressure of doing it just before you go out. Remember on some occasions you may need to ask somebody else to help you and that's ok!

- **Role play with age appropriate books.** Seek out age appropriate resources and books that will enable you to explain what is happening to you to your child. In addition to this, seek out books that help your child understand how to express their feelings and reassure them that they can talk to an adult at any time for support.

- **Avoid triggers.** As best as possible try to avoid things that make you feel unwell. You could put in place strategies to minimise your exposure to things that you know make you vomit. For example, my husband helped me by changing my daughter's nappy before going to work.

- **Remove guilt.** Mum guilt is a real feeling. It is easy to feel guilty for being unwell whilst looking after your child but always remembers that this is not your fault. Think happy thoughts that you are giving your child a sibling to play with and that this is only for a short time.

A POEM FROM THE AUTHOR

A poem from the author - written while pregnant with HG and raising a child:

Same as before... Sick as a dog
Just like before,
Worried
Just like before,
Unwanted advice,
Just like before,
Bordering depression,
Just like before.

Shock horror,
Just like before,
My body not working,
Just like before,
Maybe it won't happen they said
Just like before
Meanwhile I suffer
Just like before.

Think of the end
Just like before
But cry everyday
Just like before
Hot cold sick
Just like before
But gotta keep it in
Just like before

Are you not grateful?
Just like before
Of course it's precious
Just like before
But...Forget it
Just like before
Some words are unspoken
Just like before

Pain disappointment and happiness together
Just like before
But yet so much fear
Just like before
Was that a twinge
Just like before
Or am I paranoid?
Just like before

You carrying a child
Just like before
So buckle up and try
Just like before
The mind and body are weak
Just like before
I think I need sleep
Just like before
The hip, the lip, they all feel sick
Just like before
But dare not say too much
It's actually
Just like before.

Although this time there is a difference
Unlike before
You have someone who needs you
Unlike before
She wants her active mummy
Unlike before
Milk, food and play needed
Unlike before.

She wants to climb you and shout roar
Unlike before
Nappy changes make you vomit
Unlike before
She has needs you must meet
Unlike before
But you struggle to meet them
Unlike before

You cry for yourself and for her
Unlike before
You feel incompetent
Unlike before
You will soon have two
Unlike before
That's double blessing
Unlike before
You'll be loving two children
Unlike before
With every ounce of love in your body
Unlike before.

Final note:
So go away Hyperemesis gravidarum,
You witch
You're ruining my experience,
You're actually a witch
You come like a thief in the night
Beyond all odds
To destroy my view of the light
But one of these days
We will work out how
To decrease your movements
Because quite frankly you are foul!!!!!!!!

9

INTIMACY

For some women who suffer from HG intimacy is the last thing on their mind. It is a no go especially, when you are nauseous and depressed all at once. I mean all you do is attempt to eat, vomit and sleep. Surely the sex that caused you to be in this HG situation is not on your mind, right? WRONG!

There were days when I felt so vulnerable that a cuddle would suffice but, there were other days when having known what intimacy was and now not being able to fully take advantage of it made me sad. Yes, I was sick, but I wanted to be sexy and sick if that was even possible. Looking at my Hubby I found myself thinking, when we will ever be normal again? No matter how much he loved me or how hard I tried the headscarf, comfy clothes and miserable face never felt attractive. I began to think *'oh man this is not what he bargained for nor what he signed up for in marriage.'* I worried that I was a burden and quite frankly an inconvenience to him. I would try hard to sit up and be the usual me, but the truth was I just couldn't. I forced myself to try and cook now and then but, even that would make me feel sick! I kept thinking *'is this happening to me?'* For me to become a mother, my role as a wife became redundant.

The pressures of being an all singing, and all dancing superwoman were always weighing over me. You cook, you clean, and you are a boss in all areas, and nothing gets in your way. Well, that was the mantra often hailed. I remember the advice given by the '*aunties*' at my traditional wedding and it was '*You must feed your man well, clean the house and make sure he is not neglected otherwise, someone else would look after him for you.*' I was doing none of the above and I had no energy to worry about anything else. These ideals that I often heard '*aunties*' spew while I was growing up were so annoying, surely being a wife did not only consist of ensuring that the house was clean, husband fed and that you are always available to your husband sexually. This was an unrealistic way of living in my opinion, but that's another book for another time. Despite my own opinion on this way of thinking and knowing that I was doing nothing wrong it still kept popping up in the back of my mind. It often led to me wondering what my Hubby's Mum thought of me at the time. This followed with the constant questioning in my head: How does he feel? Am I enough? Am I doing enough? I often lay there over thinking, forgetting that my only job at this point was to stay well, healthy and alive. I was growing a little human in my belly and that was the priority.

Back to intimacy, there was a strong fear that if I allowed myself to relax in special moments, it may result in me being sick. Letting my guard down in the moment of intimacy almost felt like something I was not entitled to because of my HG condition, after all, I couldn't work, I couldn't cook, and I certainly could not feel romantic. Could I?

Words of Encouragement

The truth is there is no rule on how you are supposed to feel. Do not put any unnecessary pressure on yourself to try and do things sexually, physically and mentally that are clearly out of your capacity. This is a time where the true meaning of marriage and relationships comes to the forefront. It is not a time for you to begin beating yourself up at the possibility that your partner may go elsewhere because you are not available to him. Understand and know this that you are sick, and you are suffering from HG, it is serious and life-threatening. At this point, sex may not be a priority, and that is ok. Any person who you are committed to, love and loves you have made that commitment to you in sickness and in health. This is the sickness part therefore; your partner will need to be there for you. At the beginning stages, it is to be expected that lack of understanding and knowledge of the condition may mean that you need to give your partner a little bit more insight into how you feel. I encourage you to find at least a slither of energy just to express what you are feeling to your partner so that he can gain some understanding of what it is you're going through. That said you need to focus on reducing anxiety and any unnecessary stress.

Make the effort if and when you are feeling well enough to spend quality time with your partner. It may not be having sex or doing the things that you used to but make the best of the situation and find a way that works for you. Yes, you will not have any interesting night out pictures to post on social media, but there will be a time when you will be able to return to having another night out.

At this point in your relationship communication is vital. Allow yourself to express the feelings you have verbally to your partner. Don't expect your partner to automatically know your needs and likewise, don't assume your partner's needs. He is the father of this child; therefore, help him understand the journey that you are on by communicating how you feel. When you do this, do not expect your partner to respond in the way that you would want him to at this time as neither of you has ever experienced this before. Even if this is not your first HG pregnancy you certainly will see some differences in each pregnancy.

It is still very important that you still have alone time with your partner, even if other family members are living with you or you are getting support from people outside of your relationship. I understand that it is quite easy to just let the care that you need come from your Mum or your aunt or a friend. This may seem like the easier option, but do not isolate him. This is a different time to any time you may have experienced before so play it by ear.

10

CHILDBIRTH

I planned to have a water birth at a birthing centre as opposed to a hospital. I wanted to take videos and lots of pictures of the whole birthing experience. I also wanted to spend time in prayer and share the moment with my Mum and husband who were both my birthing partners. However, all of these dreams were shattered in both my births because my pregnancy was classed as high risk. Although HG was my biggest problem during both my pregnancies I had other issues such as obstetric cholestasis, pelvic girdle pain (which resulted in me needing to use crutches) and diabetes that developed. These issues also meant that I could not have the water birth, childbirth music, scents or affirmations that I wanted.

In addition to this, in both pregnancies I had to be induced at 38 weeks and as hard as it may be to believe the vomiting and nausea did not stop during the childbirth process. I continued to vomit up until I gave birth. HG pushed me to my limits throughout the pregnancy and it didn't spare me during Labour. I was in so much pain but that didn't matter as I was excited about the vomiting coming to an end soon after labour and the fact that I'd meet my new baby. The thought of being free from HG took away the fear of the pain and worry about whether or not I would have an epidural, gas and air or pethidine. All that mattered at the time was getting my baby out safely after months of vomiting daily.

The day before I gave birth to my daughter I remember I had been at my cousin's wedding. I could barely manage to sit straight on the chair because I kept getting feelings that I could only describe as twinges. It was unbearable but because I just wanted to be at my cousin's wedding I looked on as everyone danced. I thought about trying to move around to greet people and even dance like everyone else but, something in my body was just not allowing me. Finally I went on the dance floor and did one or two moves only to find myself retiring back to my chair to continue debating in my head whether these twinges were real or not. I had had a midwife appointment the day before and the consultant decided to do a sweep only to identify that I was one centimetre dilated so the twinges were to be expected. After such a lovely wedding we rushed home for me to rest. When we got home I continued to feel uncomfortable, but I knew I was going to be induced in less than 48 hours, so I wasn't too worried.

The pain was bad, but I was somehow managing. It was more the consistency of the pain that I was worried about as to whether or not that meant that the baby may come right then. I managed to sleep and wake up the next morning feeling brighter but still having the consistent pains. The pain got worse and at this point it had been going on for over 30 hours. I remember one of my aunt's passing by and finding me in the back room struggling with a contraction. She took one look at me and said, "You're in labour, why haven't you called your midwife?" When she said that I started to wonder why I hadn't called. I had to question myself 'Why hadn't I called the midwife to find out what to do next?' You see my whole pregnancy had been focussed around trying to keep eating, drinking and staying hydrated. While I knew contractions would come, I just assumed that I would need to be induced because that's what my consultant had planned. The idea of going into labour naturally was not something I thought was going to happen, so I dismissed the consistency of the contractions.

On instruction from my auntie we eventually called the midwife and explained to her what was going on. Even though my induction was planned for the next day the midwife asked us to come in that day. She stressed that it was important that I came in and got checked out. So, she asked us to bring everything we needed as there was a chance that I would have the baby on that day.

If I'm honest I was not nervous, and I was not scared. I didn't have any preconceptions about the labour at all. I thought about the fact that this would be the end of my HG, so I got my things together and got in the car. My Dad bid me farewell and Hubby drove to the hospital. A midwife checked me over and confirmed that I was only two centimetres dilated. Unexpectedly on arrival to the hospital having been admitted there several times I was met by an agency midwife I had never met before, she quite quickly expressed that I was not ready to give birth. She said we should go home but, as time went on she could see that I was not about to take her sending me home lightly. After all, I had been suffering for many hours. My husband also asked her to check my history thoroughly so she could see that I had a planned induction for the next day and the various challenges I had had while pregnant. It is disappointing to say but, I did a bit of name dropping about who had been involved in my care and expressed my anxiety about going home in such pain. Eventually, I was finally told that I would not be going home as it was clear that due to my other pregnancy related illnesses, the HG and the planned induction there was no longer need for me to return home.

Although I was having contractions when I went to the hospital I still needed some help and was still given the planned medication to be induced. It was very painful at this point but, again in my head I was still very focused on the HG process being over. On that night we went back and forth between contractions and pain, and I was moved from the labour ward to the delivery suite. Gas and air were my friends. I remember the doctor coming in and saying we need to *"Break your waters now so that you can progress more smoothly."* Having had my waters broken at 9:25 a.m. I was then introduced to a different agency midwife who was going to take care of me for the duration of my labour.

Once my waters were broken the midwife was quite concerned that I would no longer be able to withstand any more pain and, it would be better for me to just take an epidural to put me out of the pain. Hubby being the man that he is, rejected this immediately and challenged the midwife, he questioned her reasons for pushing me towards an epidural without consulting my birth plan. Now we all know that during labour birth plans can go completely in the bin and you just have to get through and get you and baby out safely. On this occasion, however, I was in labour and had just had my waters broken, and even though I was in pain there were other methods of pain relief that could have been explored before going to an epidural. The midwife claimed that I was nowhere near due to having this baby and therefore, if I was struggling with the pain now I would not be able to give my best when the time comes to push because I would be extremely exhausted. The midwife also expressed that if I got too far into labour I would not be able to have the epidural. If I'm honest Hubby was not happy, and he stood his ground as my Mum looked on and I could see she was thinking 'yes!' as she certainly didn't want me to have an epidural due to several stories about epidural (none of which were backed by scientific evidence). So we opted for pethidine which was given to me shortly after 10 a.m.

I remember saying to my midwife that something is happening, but she dismissed it and insisted that I was nowhere near having this baby as they had just broken your waters. She then popped out, and I immediately opened my eyes, looked at my husband and Mum and said, "Something is happening!" I felt myself rising off the bed and my legs opening without me wanting to open them, and I could not help but push. I had absolutely no control over the feelings I was getting and how my body was responding to those feelings. My Mum tried to calm me down but, again I kept emphasising that something was happening. My husband decided to look under the covers and, there she was, my daughter's head was crowning. He screamed, and then we all screamed, then he ran out into the hallway and called whoever he could see that looked like a member of staff. After all he has never delivered a baby before and he wasn't about to start now. The two people passing were students and as they entered and saw a baby's head they rushed to call for help. A doctor rushed in and delivered my baby perfectly despite not knowing anything about me.

By 10.25am my baby was out and in my arms. She was delivered by a doctor who was just passing on that ward. I remember at the point when my baby was coming out, the doctor asked what my name was.

I was overwhelmed with joy; I had a beautiful baby girl that I had spent the last 38 week thinking about. She was out, healthy, strong and had bright eyes. I knew I wanted to breastfeed but didn't know what I was doing so I just put her there anyway and hoped for the best. It was the most beautiful moment of my life and I got to share it with my Mum and my husband. The tears that flowed were for the months of sickness, and the gratitude for the beautiful baby that I had been given the honour to mother. I was overwhelmed with the fact that I didn't experience ridiculous amounts of pain or struggle to push her out. She came out when she was ready and how she wanted within an hour of my waters being broken. The pethidine hadn't set in, but I had managed somehow to do this, and she was healthy. We embraced the moment and looked at her beautiful black hair, which was full on her head, and the most gorgeous face. She was perfect. I completely blocked out all the noise and the moving around that was going on in the room. The fact that the person who delivered my baby didn't know my name and the fact that my midwife was nowhere to be seen didn't even bother me at the time. I felt blessed. I was so engrossed in looking at my gorgeous baby.

I am sure you're wondering where the midwife was. She returned to find me enjoying skin to skin with my beautiful bouncing baby girl while I looked at her wrapped up. I wish I could say I acknowledged anything that the midwife said from that point on, but I'd be lying. You see she abandoned me when I needed her because while I was telling her what my body was doing she felt she was more equipped to tell me about my own body. Quite frankly, the fact that the HG had stopped that very second and I had this beautiful baby girl on my lap left me with no feelings towards this midwife. I let her look at my baby and congratulate me just as I would anyone. I never called her up for abandoning me and I never questioned her professional judgement, which was clearly wrong at the time. I didn't have time for that because I was so happy that I was no longer being sick.

Consequently my file was updated to document that I have something called precipitate labour. This means that I can have quick labours and, if I say I'm going to push then it's probably likely that the baby is about to come. This was honoured and observed with the birth of my son. Again, the contractions started on the day that I was due to be induced. When I arrived at the hospital they didn't waste any time and I was taken straight to the delivery suite. My labour was slightly longer as from the moment my waters broke it took 4 hours for me to deliver the baby. Despite being extremely exhausted my midwife looked after me exceptionally well and did not leave my side apart from when it was time for her break. It was the most beautiful experience and again my HG stopped the day after giving birth to my son.

Words of Encouragement

I don't think you will ever meet anyone that will say they are excited for childbirth than someone who is suffering with HG. Knowing that childbirth will end the misery of vomiting every single day for months on end is overwhelming. Of course, you will have your fears and apprehensions about birth as any woman would but, the joy of no longer having to take several tablets a day and vomiting is something. That said it doesn't take away the pain that we all go through in labour nor does it take away the need for the experience to be as beautiful as possible and therefore, I offer these encouragements:

- Pack your maternity bag as any pregnant woman would but, make sure to include everything you need that helps you with your HG. The fact that you're in labour doesn't mean that you won't need these things. Speak to the staff on the ward and tell them what you need. Do not be shy to ask for things that you require to make you just that little bit more comfortable. For example I desperately wanted ice which they found for me.

- Be prepared for the possibility that you may not stop vomiting immediately after giving birth. After I gave birth to my daughter I stopped vomiting but, with my son I didn't stop until the day after he was born. I was overwhelmed by the fact that I was no longer being sick and started to think about eating everything all at once but, go easy on yourself. You spent several weeks vomiting, so enjoy your food but take time to allow yourself to adjust.

- Be sure that you have people who will advocate for you during labour. The reason I say this is because for example, black women are five times more likely to die in childbirth. Professionals may brush over some of your symptoms or expect you to manage them due to their stereotypes of the type of person you may be. For this reason it is crucial that you have people with you that can stand up for you and protect you if this does happen.

I always wanted my Mum to be present during my labour, so I am glad that she was able to be there for both. My mother is very prayerful and has always been my rock, but she is not a person who will have any form of confrontation or stand up against a professional. This is something that we see in the older generation as they trust in professional guidance and instructions as we should. However, it is extremely important that if you are unsure about something or think that something is not right you question and challenge it. This is the role my husband took in the labour room. For him to do this he needed to be aware of what I wanted and what I didn't want so make sure you have those conversations before you go to the labour room. This prepares you for any scenario where you are unable to advocate for yourself.

11

YOUR MENTAL WELLBEING AFTER BIRTH

After having the babies you would think my world would return to normal and that I would return to being confident and happy but that has not been the case. It was not until I attended an event hosted by a friend on perinatal and postnatal depression that I realised that I was suffering from post-traumatic stress disorder (PTSD). I remember listening to a speaker talk about PTSD in relation to birth traumas. The emphasis was on going into labour, and having a really traumatic experience that has lasting effects on the mother. One lady talked about her pregnancy and the impact that the trauma in her pregnancy had on her. Then it dawned on me, I was still being affected by my HG experiences.

A symptom that I almost didn't notice was my anxiety about having an unplanned pregnancy or another pregnancy at all. Seeing the impact my previous pregnancies had had on me, the family, my job and finances really made me conscious that trying to do that again with two children under five would be extremely difficult. I was aware that there is a chance that I may get HG again, so I had it in my head that if I ever considered having another child it would be controlled and I would have live-in help in order to support me. This went from a thought at the back of my mind to a continuous worry. Eventually, it became overwhelming especially when the 'aunties' would say I should go for one more as though it was as easy as that. I would find myself explaining that HG does not permit me to make such rash decisions.

Even though I was using contraception the fears of falling pregnant outside of this plan meant that before my menstrual cycle I would be worried and monitor my period calendar continuously. It was not until I had the intrauterine device (coil) fitted that I became a little more relaxed but, even then people's jokes about me being pregnant got to me. I would find myself going to several lengths to convince myself and them that I wasn't. Anxiety.

If ever I felt unwell and it included nausea or vomiting I would always put it down to me possibly being pregnant, and result in me getting into a state of panic. Vomiting gave me flashbacks of how I would vomit during my pregnancy. It almost felt like even celibacy would not stop me from attributing all vomiting to pregnancy. I also found that I could vomit quite easily. A bad smell, bad pain or even hunger could make me feel nauseous or vomit.

Wanting more children is something that I stopped feeling entitled to due to the fact that several people passed comments like "Your pregnancies are difficult, so don't do it to yourself". This made me feel as though getting pregnant again would not be received well by the people around me. Bearing in mind that I genuinely needed support to get through my HG.

I noticed that all of my worrying began to take over me and I often worried about things that others would say are not that deep. I felt like my HG had put me under scrutiny for the whole 38 weeks as a result I became a lot more indecisive and thought a lot deeper into the opinions of others about me. Although I know that HG was not my fault I still blamed myself. I regretted not standing up to people who made snide comments that left me feeling down during my pregnancy. Of course, I could do nothing about now.

Every area of my life started to show cracks and myself belief was dwindling. I would constantly over think most things. The once confident person I knew myself to be would cry, panic and worry easily. The final straw was when I began looking for employment; initially I had been looking for roles that involved little responsibility despite my skills and qualifications. I considered the potential of another child in a particular type of role and the thought alone made me nervous. Anxiety.

I sat in the event about perinatal and postnatal depression and realised I was potentially suffering with something off the back of my experiences with HG. I sought advice from one of the speakers at the event and she confirmed my concerns that I would need to get some help dealing with the experiences I had in relation to HG. I felt so empowered and contacted a therapist the next week.

When I was finally allocated my therapist who was a man and I immediately said to the counselling allocations manager that I would prefer a female due to the nature of my experience. Clearly I had gotten it all wrong because the counselling manager explained to me that a male or woman would be required to listen to my concerns regardless and she encouraged me to give my therapist a try which I did. When I told family and friends that I was preparing to start therapy it was met with mixed emotions. On one hand it was as my friends were relieved that I was finally going to free myself from the struggle I kept having with anxiety. Unlike some who were more traditional were confused as to why I needed therapy. The thing is therapy is a personal thing so why did I tell them in the first place – self-doubt. I wanted validation that I was taking the right step towards reducing my feelings of anxiety but this in actual fact was no body's business or problem. These were fears deep rooted inside me and I knew I didn't want them to remain.

I liked my therapist; he was exceptionally attentive and even went on to research HG in depth. My therapist had no preconceptions of HG in relation to regular NVP. I remember explaining to my therapist that I can barely remember things that had happened in the first six months of my child's life because I was continuously worrying about things. When he asked me to explore what I was worried about I was able to really understand all the different things that had happened or contributed to my lack of memory. It wasn't a pleasant feeling because I had to look at videos and pictures to remind myself of some of the stages of my son's first year of life.

My therapy went deep and made me consider the deep rooted reasons why I didn't want to ever feel like a burden to people and why I was a 'people-pleaser'. The sessions really helped me to remove the layers of negative comments that had been placed on me during my pregnancies and also help me to begin to deal with my own trauma from the impact of HG.

Words of Encouragement

It is important to acknowledge the fact that you have experienced something that is extremely traumatic. You should get help or find methods to deal with the scars that remain. Therapy offers a very good source of support where you can gain access to a safe and non-judgemental space to share your thoughts and explore your experiences.

Postnatal depression or PTSD can show itself in various ways. You may feel very low or become very anxious; do not ignore your feelings as there is support out there.

Postnatal depression can impact the way you bond with your baby after birth. PTSD can lead to you experiencing panic attacks, flashbacks and even find yourself avoiding certain foods or places due to the reminder of a traumatic part of your pregnancy. Whilst they are both common after HG, support that is specific to your individual needs and concerns is available. Speak to your GP and request a referral to the postnatal mental health teams. I need to stress that at this point the 'aunties' will come and tell you how bad it was in their day, and how there was not time for postnatal depression in their day. That's fine for them but, this is about you and your needs, so don't spend time telling people who are not helping you your problem.

Finally join your fellow HG survivors by spreading awareness of HG through your story building awareness within our communities.

A LETTER FROM MY HUSBAND

Dear Reader,

I didn't see this coming, I never thought I would have the opportunity to talk about the impact that my wife's pregnancy experiences had on me. During her pregnancies, she was diagnosed with HG, which physically and mentally affected her. You'd think that as a man I wouldn't have been affected, but as a committed husband, I experienced every bit of what she was going through.

After we got married, it took a while before my wife became pregnant, the day she broke the news to me I was so happy, that to celebrate I would have bought her the whole world if I could. The real experience started at our first midwife appointment, and I didn't want to miss any part of the journey so I made the effort to adjust my work schedule in order to always be present.

When the symptoms of HG started creeping in, initially I thought it was morning sickness so I didn't give it much thought. As time went on it started getting worse and that is when I learnt that there was something called Hyperemesis Gravidarum. I watched helplessly as my wife worked hard to persevere through her pregnancy with the symptoms of HG, unfortunately this pregnancy resulted in a miscarriage. I will never forget that night.

When my wife became pregnant for the second time, the thought and the experience from the miscarriage was still fresh in my mind. So, when she told me that she was pregnant, initially I didn't know what to feel, yes I wanted a baby so bad but I was worried about her. People around you think that it's all about getting pregnant, but for us being pregnant was very challenging because of HG.

I experienced anxiety and I found myself crying at random times when no one was around. You know as men it is believed that we are "macho" so men don't cry. So I would wipe my tears and push on.

It was extremely important that we were surrounded by supportive family and friends to remind us that "it shall be well" and to help us through the difficult times especially as I was still working. If I'm honest the sound of her vomiting and us being late to places due to her vomiting almost became normal. Attending events alone was not fun and I was often present but spent a lot of time on the phone to my wife showing her what was going on via video call.

I had to become more domesticated around the house but I knew it was never as good as how she would have done it herself. I had to learn how to do things to her standard. I felt pressure as she looked on and often I would ask her to tell me the right way to do all that she usually did without any complaint. I had to learn how to grill Salmon in the way she liked otherwise one mistake would mean she wouldn't eat it at all.

As a healthcare professional, I worked in a hospital during the time my wife suffered from HG, so I had experienced being around sick people. After a day at work I felt like I was going from one ward of patients and coming home to what was almost like another patient. It was very tiring and hard. I felt like I had no choice but to not think about myself and focus on being there for my wife. I would clean her sick and remove anything that she said made her feel sick just to ease her pressure. I had to be quick on my feet because if she said the sickness was coming it really was, and I often had to pull over in the most random places to accommodate this. Yes, it did get frustrating but I had no choice. My wife was sick.

My wife is my rock and therefore, seeing her so poorly left me vulnerable. She is my support system. No matter how much I tried to explain it to my male friends and even my Mum who lives in Ghana no one really understood the full impact of HG, not to forget that HG is not the only thing that happens whilst a woman is pregnant. My sister has five children and never experienced this so it was harder to explain to my family back home. So, they panicked every time she was admitted to get fluids.

Looking back on it, it would have been better for me to have someone to talk to after our HG journey and drop the stigma that men have to be strong and carry everyone around them. HG affects men emotionally. Men are often expected to show less emotion in difficult times and in the circumstances you may need to be strong for her but, it is important that you find your own outlet. This will enable you to be your best for her.

I am grateful to God for blessing us with our beautiful children and to my wife for remaining strong and enduring such difficulties. I am so proud that she is now helping others through what is one of the most challenging things I think anyone can experience.

Yours sincerely,

K. Buabeng

LETTERS FROM SURVIVORS

Dear Reader,

My name is Cyndy and I am proud to say I am a Survivor or Hyperemesis Gravidurum. I survived mentally, physically and emotionally. Some may see HG as just severe morning sickness, which is a normal part of pregnancy, but it isn't that easy. It is much more than that. What it does to you mentally, emotionally and physically without the support can have some long-lasting effects.

For both my pregnancies I had HG, however, for my daughter, I really went through it. I was admitted to the hospital more times than I could count, for day stays to weeklong stays.

Imagine vomiting and urinating yourself at the same time because your whole body is in shock and cannot function properly. I was vomiting so much that all that was coming out was bile on a daily basis, imagine vomiting so much you really question whether you could do this!

What really affected me, was people saying, just eat a little, so the baby can get some food. You know you're eating for two, if you don't eat the baby will not survive. In my mind I felt like because I could not eat, I was not being a good mother and I was killing my child before she was even born. I could not eat or even drink water... simple water. I lost so much weight and I became so dehydrated my skin started changing colour. I really did feel inadequate and I felt like I was not providing the nutrition's my baby needed. I was afraid, and I just could not bring myself to explain what I was going through. I just wished that there was a service with survivors who could encourage me through this struggle at the time.

For anyone suffering from HG, I want to say, just keep pushing forward and do not suffer alone, speak with someone because doing this alone with no one who understands can affect your mental health. I would also like to emphasise that eating for two is a MYTH... It does not mean double your portions.

You're a Super Mum and you're doing the best that you can... which is more than enough.

Yours sincerely,

Cyndy Kowah,
MUA and Founder of Ava Rhyan

Dear Reader,

At six weeks I felt incredibly nauseous and was struggling to eat and keep down any foods or liquids without vomiting. As a Nurse and Health Visitor, I knew this was not good. I went to the GP and felt like my condition wasn't being taken seriously even though I informed them that I had a family history of Hyperemesis Gravidarum. This continued at the 8 weeks pregnancy mark, so I contacted my GP and was immediately brought in for an emergency appointment. After my check-up, I was sent straight to the Emergency Department because I was severely dehydrated and weak. I stayed there all night and was put on fluids. I was informed that I was getting the best form of medication for my condition, and things should improve within a week. Friends and family gave advice on things that worked for them, or from what they read, such as trying foods with ginger, which I tried, but as mentioned before, I couldn't keep it down. By week 16 I had been admitted four times to take fluids overnight. I would also vomit severely 10-15 times a day, although I wasn't eating anything, so for the most part, it was my stomach acids that were being regurgitated.

I had to tell colleagues, friends and family I was pregnant, much earlier than I would have liked, as I was so severely ill and often bed-bound, and not able to speak to anyone. I was unable to enjoy the pregnancy like I would have hoped to and just wanted it to end so that I could feel better again. I really did not know how I would manage like this as I got older, as I did want more children down the line. Fortunately, I had a supportive husband, who was able to help me. But I felt bad, as it was impacting him and his work. As he would have to help me move around and take me to hospital, whilst trying to attend work meetings and carry out presentations.

By week 19, I began to feel a lot better and had what I imagined regular morning sickness felt like. However, I had to take multiple medications throughout the day and night, but I was able to walk around now and begin to enjoy my pregnancy, although the sickness was still there, it was not as severe as in the early stages. I was able to explain to my employers in great detail what I was experiencing, and they were supportive and allowed me to reduce my hours, come in late and accommodated me and my work schedule around the latter part of the pregnancy.

By the 40th week, I went into labour for 36 hours and gave birth to a beautiful healthy baby boy. To this day, I think the labour was much easier than any of the pregnancy and severe sickness I felt from HG. I would like another baby, but I am scared to go through that experience again, with the additional responsibility of a child to care for at the same time.

Just because you are ill now, doesn't mean you won't get better throughout the pregnancy. You will get through it. Getting the right medication early, makes a difference and having at least one supportive and understanding person helps a lot.

Yours sincerely,

Krystal Mesmain BSc (Hons), BSc (Hons), PGDip, RGN, SCPHN.HV, V100
Specialist Health Visitor in Perinatal and Infant Mental Health

Dear Reader,

I was about seven weeks pregnant when I started showing the symptoms of HG. I remember standing up, and then I suddenly retched. I was full of shock. I looked at my husband with wide eyes, and I took his advice to go to the toilet but I didn't make the ten or so steps before I vomited again.

The prescribed antiemetic medicine kind of worked, but taking it resulted in drowsiness and me being knocked out for twenty minutes. It was either I was nauseous or just passed out. The resulting exhaustion was deliberating, I remember being comatose in my car after an episode. Many a time HG made me seriously question whether I was capable of pregnancy and motherhood. After years of extensive fertility treatment I was shocked that pregnancy could make me feel so broken, I thought it was behind me now.

I felt so exhausted by the time I had my nine weeks scan that my first thought when I saw my long awaited miracle baby on the screen was 'You little sod.' Even in that moment I was struggling to house my stomach contents, so much so that I could barely hear what the sonographer was saying. The sickness hampered everything, as trying not to vomit became a daily task. It was so bad that I nearly killed myself due to suddenly projectile vomiting while driving at 50mph in the middle lane. Luckily the A406 being randomly quiet that day saved me as I dangerously swerved and halted.

On the upside, I made friends with a station guard who would keep me company on the platform while I spewed into my commuter sick bag. The vomiting only stopped when I reached the six months mark and that is when I began to fully enjoy the pregnancy. The nausea reduced but it lasted until birth. Obviously it was all worth it and I would do it again in a heartbeat. Though I'm sad that I can never look a pickled onion Monster Munch in the eye without the taste of bile in my throat.

Yours sincerely,

Charlene Perrier,
HG Survivor

Dear Reader,

Whenever I think back to my pregnancy it never really fills me with delight as it was one of the hardest things I've ever encountered. I was surprised to find out that I was pregnant, and that at that point I was already three weeks gone. It was really early in my pregnancy journey, but I was vomiting everywhere and all the time. I quickly got signed off work at about 8 weeks and Hubby and I decided that I should just quit and focus on the new chapter. I always thank God for blessing me with such an amazing husband especially during what felt like a hard and lonely season. I couldn't explain to anyone why I was constantly throwing up, and though my midwife offered six different types of antiemetic tablets I still kept vomiting. I tried all six and I couldn't hold any food down. As a result, it became a regular visit to the hospital so that I could receive some fluids and even then I would still vomit. I was 59kg pre-pregnancy and dropped to 49kg during my pregnancy. I was literally just a bump. I remember the constant tips on how to gain more weight. Honestly, if I could add a kg for every time someone advised me to try ginger or drink tea, maybe I would have looked like a normal pregnant woman.

I spent the majority of my pregnancy in bed because I couldn't even stand the smell of the kitchen. It was extremely lonely, as Hubby was at work and I'm the first in my friendship group to have a baby. I recall my husband coming home to shower me because of a lack of energy to even get up. It was hard is an understatement. He is the only one who understands why I tend to say I'm not ready to have another nor do I know if I want to. I struggled to talk to Asaiah, my daughter, during the pregnancy because firstly, I was so surprised, and secondly, I was so weak in my body then, thirdly I was terrified. What if this pregnancy was going to kill me? I'm not exaggerating but maybe the hormones really took their toll on me. I wouldn't change my pregnancy for anything. It's made me super strong and I love my daughter. I wish, however, that there was an increase of awareness of Hyperemesis so that people can be a little more understanding when a woman tells you this is what she's going through.

Yours sincerely,

Ashley Nkosana,
Founder of Self Love Journeys

ABOUT THE AUTHOR

ABOUT THE AUTHOR

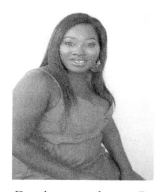

Multi-award winning Rachael Buabeng is a wife, mother, step-mother, author of Kofi and Adjoa Stories and the founder of Mummy's Day Out Ltd.

Rachael grew up in East London to Ghanaian born parents who coincidentally are also called Kofi and Adjoa as are her children. She has always been passionate about children's learning and development which led her to study and graduate with a Business and Child Development degree. Rachael later went on to become a qualified teacher delivering various subjects; specialising in childcare and education. Now Rachael juggles motherhood and her businesses.

Mummy's Day Out brings mothers together to reduce isolation and offers them the opportunity to socialise with like-minded mothers, with their children in tow. The events aim to inspire, encourage and empower women on their motherhood journey.

Rachael was inspired by her children to begin to write children's books as she wanted to capture their experiences and to ensure that they could see themselves represented in the books they read.

Rachael now continues to be a keynote speaker locally and internationally and uses her social media platforms to encourage mothers on their motherhood journey. After extremely difficult pregnancies Rachael identified a lack of awareness of HG generally but more so in the BAME community which inspired her to write this book. She now advocates for HG survivors by sharing her own extreme experiences of adversity as a mother to encourage others. Rachael provides support across her social media platforms which she uses to respond to mothers needs/interests and shed light on issues relating to motherhood.

To find out more about the author and her books, visit:
www.rachaelbuabeng.com

Or to contact her please email:
info@rachaelbuabeng.com

Printed in Great Britain
by Amazon